feel *good* AGAIN

feel
good
AGAIN

*A Game-Changing Guide
to Creating Wellness,
Energy, Joy and
an Enthusiasm for Life*

Linda Goggin, MD

NEW YORK

NASHVILLE • MELBOURNE • VANCOUVER

feel *good* AGAIN
A Game-Changing Guide to Creating Wellness, Energy, Joy and an Enthusiasm for Life

Published in New York, New York, by Morgan James Publishing in partnership with Difference Press. Morgan James is a trademark of Morgan James, LLC. www.MorganJamesPublishing.com

The Morgan James Speakers Group can bring authors to your live event. For more information or to book an event visit The Morgan James Speakers Group at www.TheMorganJamesSpeakersGroup.com.

ISBN 978-1-68350-563-1 paperback
ISBN 978-1-68350-564-8 eBook
Library of Congress Control Number: 2017906654

Cover Design by:
Rachel Lopez
www.r2cdesign.com

Interior Design by:
Bonnie Bushman
The Whole Caboodle Graphic Design

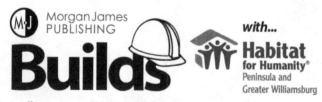

In an effort to support local communities, raise awareness and funds, Morgan James Publishing donates a percentage of all book sales for the life of each book to Habitat for Humanity Peninsula and Greater Williamsburg.

Get involved today! Visit
www.MorganJamesBuilds.com

Dedication

Colin Warner Henry Goggin
All my love and a gazillion hugs for all your support!

Charlie, Zoe, and Henry
I love you all to the end of the Universe and back!

Table of Contents

Foreword

Who doesn't want to feel good? ...Nobody! That's why I was so pleased when Dr. Linda Goggin asked me to read her new book, *Feel Good Again*. You will love her fresh perspective and lively tone as she serves up a fun, readable account of the basics of functional medicine and how you can apply these principles in your life with great results. Making habit change *fun* is the best way to make habit change easy and permanent... that is exactly what Dr. Goggin gives you.

As an educator for the Institute for Functional Medicine my prime goal is to teach practitioners how to guide their patients in the use of nutrition and lifestyle change to bring about revolutionary shifts in personal wellness. When patients begin to actively advocate for their own health, many find themselves in the office of a Functional Medicine provider, hoping to find answers, direction, and affirmation that personal health revolution is truly possible. The Functional Medicine paradigm rekindles hope and offers personalized paths to vitality. However, reclaiming wellness requires patience, persistence, and effort, with the deepest challenge being self-motivation after the novelty of the "latest, greatest program" wears off. New ways of eating must be healing, not depriving; new habits must energize instead of deplete, and each person has to find those positive motivating ideas that continue to inspire through the wellness journey. In *Feel Good Again* Dr. Goggin leads the reader to look within and find their own source of power for change while turning the work into a game. When innovative thinkers like Dr. Goggin take the time to share ideas and expertise we can expect nothing less than a revolution in the country's health status.

Today's health care is in crisis. Providers find themselves frustrated with the conundrum of how to help people make dramatic change in their lives within the span of a brief visit. We need more voices to speak out and *advocate* for the power of lifestyle medicine because these principles give people personal control over their health. I congratulate Dr. Goggin on contributing to the growing body of work devoted towards helping people help themselves. Add *Feel Good Again* to the list of must-reads for those seeking vibrant health through joyous, creative mastery of self!

Tom Malterre, MS, CN

Author of *The Elimination Diet* and *The Whole Life Nutrition Cookbook*

Introduction

"Doctor, I Feel Terrible…"

Carol had seen a lot of doctors on her journey to figuring out what the heck was wrong and why she was feeling so terrible. Apparently all her lab work was "fine," and she should get a little more exercise and eat right. She now possessed quite a few handouts—nutrition and exercise tips—and some whopping big bills. Some visits, she left feeling slightly embarrassed, as though she was complaining of nothing and she should just suck it up. But how could the overwhelming fatigue, memory issues, lack of motivation, joint pains, and headaches be nothing? She wondered if she would ever feel better; it simply didn't make sense to her. She was smart, had read a lot of self-help books about health, and had gathered many "tools for success." For some reason she found herself unable to follow through on many of these things, though, partly because she was having a hard time just making sure everybody in her family got where they needed to go on a daily basis.

Who really has time for self-care anyway?! Before, when she felt well, juggling it all was simple. But in the midst of deep fatigue and depression, sometimes just getting out of bed was hard. Not wanting to give up, she went to the next best thing to a doctor: Google. She typed in her symptoms. Headache, fatigue, bloating, hot flashes, swelling in her feet, foggy brain, dizziness, memory problems, depression, anxiety, stomach problems…. The list went on. Dr. Google just about pronounced her dead. Honestly, she had all the biggies. Multiple sclerosis, cancer of various types, degenerative neurological disease. She was going to die. Just as she was about to close the laptop in frustration, an entry caught her eye about a different way to evaluate patients by looking for the root cause of symptoms. She clicked on the link to find out more.

Hope for Doctors and Patients Alike

Opening that link opened Carol's eyes, and what she read gave her hope. She read about a new cutting-edge style of medical practice called functional medicine. A physician who takes the time to explore this new perspective can also experience a similar sense of hope: hope that medicine can once again become the sleuthing adventure they passionately described to their families as a medical student, hope of helping people who feel bad and for whom no treatment might have been previously identified, and hope that they might reclaim the fun of doctoring.

I used to run on an office-based hamster wheel, seeing 20-25 patients a day and often finding myself with a complex individual in front of me and two more waiting in other examination rooms. I wanted each patient to feel cared for and understood, and I wanted to be able to give the best information to all my clients. Handouts or tip sheets were sometimes the best I could muster. People like Carol would bring in a long list of complaints and have normal lab work; from a conventional standpoint,

I could offer little in the way of treatment. Certainly I wanted them to feel better, so I gave them lifestyle advice and symptomatic therapy. But actually reversing those nagging, persistent life-sucking symptoms like aching, fatigue, headaches, brain fog, depression, and anxiety seemed virtually impossible. Just when I was considering stepping off that wheel of purgatory into a nice barista job (where surely I could always serve up the right suds), along came functional medicine.

Functional medicine looks at each person uniquely in an effort to identify the root cause of symptoms. The term "functional" refers to basic changes in how well our bodily processes work. When these processes don't work, people get symptoms that, if left unchecked, will progress to chronic diseases. That's when you start to see abnormal lab values, and when many physicians pull out their prescription pad. As a functional medicine physician, my focus is on helping my patients identify what is making them feel sick—could be too much of something, too little of something, maybe a hormonal imbalance, perhaps a chronic viral infection—then we work on correcting imbalances, making sure each person's body has all the building blocks and essential nutrients for keeping the balls in the air, and we introduce lifestyle changes, nutritional support, and health habits that can totally revolutionize an individual's life. The goal is not suppression of symptoms, but removing the cause of the symptoms so that they resolve naturally. We are not just going for "better;" we go for the glow.

Carol's Metamorphosis

How does someone with so many symptoms find their way back to vibrant health? In functional medicine, we begin by taking an initial "snapshot with a microscope," a detailed look at the whole person, including life history and major events, health habits and routines, and investigation into their diet, support systems, and environment, along with more specific nutritional, genetic, and stool testing in the search for the root cause of the symptoms. Then we develop a plan for transformation.

Carol discovered that she lacked some vital nutrients her body needed to feel well, and an elimination diet uncovered food sensitivities that she never imagined were problems. We boosted her diet with powerful food medicine, and eliminated wicked little sabotaging foods that were making her feel like she was encased in cement and covered with chocolate frosting. Within a couple of weeks, she felt as though the fog had lifted, and her headaches had diminished in frequency by 75%.

This is what happens when we let food be our medicine; it doesn't usually take very long to see the changes. The nice thing about these basic interventions? You *don't* need a doctor to do a lot of this. Carol noticed dramatic shifts in her body over the next several weeks.

Then came the time when she started to lose momentum with the changes that she had made. "I felt as though the same old thing was starting to happen to me; I tried something for a little while and felt better, but it was hard to keep it up," she said. That's when we added the *secret sauce*. When Carol started to shake this mystery ingredient over her whole day, her life transformed.

Can you relate to Carol? Do you have multiple aggravating or debilitating symptoms or medical challenges? It could be time to find the root cause of your symptoms and shake a little of the secret sauce on you!

Doing the Right Thing for More Than a Month or Two Is Hard

How I wish I could rewind and use my current methods on previous clients! I remember feeling immense frustration with my limited toolbox when someone came to my office feeling bad and had normal lab work. Fortunately, medicine's renaissance approaches fast, and it brings fresh new approaches to caring for patients. As described in James Maskell's book, *The Evolution of Medicine*, doctors are going to have to focus on keeping people well instead of "keeping 'em coming back." This demands a deeper understanding of what creates vibrant health for each individual.

New tools such as genetically informed medical and nutritional recommendations, appreciation of and engagement with people's microbiome (our individual and highly personal entourage of bacteria), surveying for and eliminating substances with toxic potential, modalities that keep the intestinal lining happily protecting the body from inflammation, lifestyle medicine to destress and natural means to alter hormones—wow! Exciting stuff! The explosion of information coming out in so many different yet related fields makes keeping up with the most current research difficult for the typical busy physician. Additionally, it takes about 10-15 years for new information to make it into published guidelines that physicians often rely on for practice guidance. This can make figuring out whose information to believe difficult. As a whole, the health system will have to become more effective at creating individualized health prescriptions for people. Personalized medicine or not, it won't matter if we can't motivate people to do the right thing for more than a month. It is much easier to do what have always done—creatures of habit, we are.

"It's Like I Can Never Wake Up"

Chase was a star athlete in high school and went on to play college football. He needed help with the extra 30 pounds that had been lingering around his middle for the past several years along with an overwhelming sense of fatigue. "When morning comes I can never wake up," he said. "When it comes to multi-tasking, I'm not even able to chew gum and walk, and it feels like my thoughts are being poled down the river by an ancient man with a long white beard who is taking his own sweet time. I'm trying to eat a healthy diet, but I still feel hungry all the time."

Like Carol, Chase had problems with his stomach, unpredictable bloating and diarrhea that at times kept him from enjoying social events. He, too, had been to his primary care physician, who had checked some labs, including a complete blood count, run a metabolic panel, and done basic thyroid tests, but had found everything to be normal. The doctor had recommended weight loss.

When people come to see me, we do a lot of digging to figure out where they are in terms of all their habits, nutrition, stress and emotional health, support systems, exercise… that's functional medicine. Mining Chase's history meant him keeping a detailed journal evaluating everything that went in his mouth, and, at our end, running a complete thyroid panel as well as a genetic panel to evaluate for common problematic variations that are amenable to support with nutrients.

We found that he did indeed have a thyroid issue, as well as digestive issues that were affecting his ability to feel good and lose weight. I put him on a diet that supports the thyroid, used individualized supplements that were dictated by tiny variations in his genetics called SNPs (single nucleotide polymorphisms), and helped him focus on bringing his stress level down. Almost magically (especially to Chase), he felt much better in a few months and was back to a healthy weight. But as you know if you have tried to do a new program, then came the hard part. How to keep the momentum going after the emergency is over? Chase, too, needed some of my *special sauce*.

Could This Be Something Serious?

Like most people, Chase spent time on the internet trying to self-diagnose. The problem is, people rarely hit the nail on the head. More often than not, their research only makes them worry that there may be something "bad wrong." After all, they have a lot of symptoms. How can we make sure that it's not anything that could be immediately life-threatening?

A good physical examination and basic lab work rule out most health problems that require immediate acute care. In general, conventional physicians do a great job giving reassurance in this manner. But the problem is, you still feel bad, sad, and all-around tired. These are signs of chronic inflammation; inflammation causes lots of symptoms, but does not yet show up as abnormal lab work on basic panels such as complete blood count, metabolic panel, and TSH (Thyroid Stimulating Hormone)—the ones your doctor would typically order. That said, seeing a healthcare practitioner for a checkup to confirm that you do not have any life-threatening conditions is still a good idea. Most people have already done this by the time they come to see a functional medicine doctor, looking for answers as to why they still feel bad.

With issues like these, the conventional toolkit is limited. Current medical training is expanding to include new modalities; evidence-based nutrition, genomics, and personalized medicine gain footholds daily. Advances in our understanding of how our genes play into individual nutrient needs, that small variations in our genetics alter how we metabolize medications and toxins, and the interplay between our resident bacteria (our "microbiome"), our brain, and our immune system—all these herald a revolution in the way we evaluate and diagnose individuals.

Medical research involves finding a group of people who share the same characteristics and then splitting them into several groups, some of whom receive a certain treatment while others do not. The more we understand how unique each person is—their microbiome, genetic fingerprint, ability to detox, the effect that food and activity has on gene expression—the harder it will be to *truly* find a "matched cohort," i.e., a bunch of folks that have similar metabolic systems. Sure, we look similar on the outside… arms, legs, schnoz, and all. What matters is on the inside. We are snowflakes, and that makes meaningful research even more of a challenge.

Breakthroughs are coming, but traditional medicine has been so focused on finding a pill to reverse symptoms that it has downplayed the huge effect a person's lifestyle, emotions, and exposures have on their health. These days, people go to the doctor hoping for a quick fix. Unfortunately, there's no pill for inflammation and subsequent chronic disease.

Reversing Inflammation, Reversing Symptoms, Reversing Diabetes

I want my sweeties—Charlie, Henry and Zoe—to grow up feeling awesome and to be able to avoid the doctor's office when they're in their adulthood. As a mom and a doctor, the prediction that one third of today's children will end up with diabetes and that their generation will have a shorter lifespan freaks me out. There has to be a way for each of us to personally shift as well as empower world culture to do the same! The countries to whom we have exported the standard American diet are seeing the same rise in chronic illness that we're registering in the US. As research brings us more information on the big diseases that make us feel bad and eventually kill us, such as high blood pressure, heart attacks, cancers, diabetes, and autoimmune disorders, the ties to inflammation become obvious.

Inflammation is our body's response when it feels under attack, like the sounding of an alarm, and it can come from many potential sources. When this occurs over years, the impact is significant. Among the variables that lead to inflammation, what we eat figures in prominently, as well as chronic infections, poor sleep, lack of exercise, stress, lack of meaningful relationships, and toxic exposures. Nutrition, sleep, exercise, friends, clean air and water—sound familiar? Right. Grandma told us we needed this stuff. And these are within our power to change. Easy to say, harder to do. Ever tried to change a deeply ingrained habit? At first it's not too hard, and then, somehow, we find ourselves sneaking back to the fridge at 3 am. Pretty familiar song.

In my medical practice, I recognize that what my clients need, more than the medications I can prescribe, is better food, fewer toxic exposures, less stress, more fun, and a solid way to change their habits for good. As people remove food that causes inflammation and boost their nutrition by eating clean, nutrient-dense foods, their symptoms get better. If they're able to keep walking the walk for the long haul, they will not only live longer, but their body will be working better during that time. Everyone is scared of dying, but what's even worse is to have 20 or 30 years at the end of your life where you feel like total hell. So raise your kombucha glass high; here's to evolution.

Pushing Through the Wall After Initial Change

It's no fun to be stuck—actually, it's miserable, and that's really what I see as a huge problem for most of my clients. Most are feeling bad enough that they are very motivated for short-term intervention. However, once the emergency is over and they feel a little better, they tend to drift back to "old ways." Frankly, I'm describing myself here also. I used to find developing and maintaining new habits extremely difficult. When I discovered the secret to deep, permanent health evolution, I wanted to tell every person I met. It's simple and extremely powerful.

Based upon scientific research, this big reveal is something your kids could have told you: it just has to be fun, like a hobby; it needs to be a game. The new activity or habit must be *more appealing* than the old ways, *even when you're being taunted by obstacles.* There are plenty of books that can give you solid advice on the steps to take to feel better. I see the true problem as implementation. Sure, I can read a book and recognize that I should follow the "program." But how do I make myself want to do it after I feel a little bit better? I want to keep evolving, and I know you do, too.

Almost no one can buy into doing something over the long haul simply because someone else told them to do it. We like control. We may be rebels. We have cherished habits that we really, really, really can't give up. Getting out of our routines can be uncomfortable, and people naturally drift back to doing the things that they have done repetitively. This goes for habits of thought, emotions, actions, relationship patterns, you name it. So what's the hack? How do we get past our basic nature, when our basic nature is pulling us to comfort and familiarity? Stretching our edges is, in a word, uncomfortable. Why is it that when I need to sit down and apply myself to a task, I find myself cleaning the kitchen? Habit. Something I know how to do. It takes my anxiety level down. The option of applying myself to this new task is not as appealing or comforting, and certainly not as fun to me as getting a clean kitchen.

Let's run down a list of things that we might want to add into our lives to make us healthier and happier: exercise, healthy cooking, playing Candy Crush Saga—wait a minute…. Playing Candy Crush Saga? That's not on most "healthy and happy" lists. That sounds kind of fun, and possibly better than going on a run! Wouldn't it be wonderful if we could capture the fun of a game in our quest to build a healthy body, mind, and spirit? What if we could make the idea of a run give us the same charge as playing a game?

You may have heard about the idea of "gamification," or turning drudgery and stuff you don't want to do into a game. Mary Poppins, the pioneer in gamification, said it first: "In every job that must be done, there is an element of fun. Find the fun, and *snap!* The job's a game!" Flash forward a few decades, and gamification is now all the rage.

Medicine needs to jump on and ride this wave. As a physician, I feel that my main mission is to help people find a way to make permanent changes in their health habits to take their wellness to a higher level. As a mom, I want my children to turn into healthy adults and let go of the pizza, already! These are one and the same. Kids given proper guidance will naturally cycle upward in terms of their health habits. Do you remember when you started to pick up some healthy habits as a teenager, or as a young adult? The hard part is consistently cycling upward, and that's what this book is meant to do. You enter the cycle of change wherever you are at this moment without apologies, with full acceptance, and you level up to a higher plane from there.

Let's plan on getting you feeling better in two months. Find your new set point. Live at your new set point and then let's keep gradually moving toward our higher self, toward full, vibrant wellness. We want to keep your health revolution going. Imagine gliding up a spiral, with each loop feeling a little better. Feeling more of your power. Take my hand, let's evolve now!

So what makes this different? Why is this more than just a silly book on health habits that you read for a weekend and lose under the couch? Enter *secret sauce*! The secret sauce is in making changing your health habits *fun*. Turning daunting tasks into games and breaking huge projects into tiny, manageable steps makes the impossible possible. Grab a friend, because it's more fun with a buddy. This concept is backed by research; studies on gameplay reveal that the mental boost we get when we play a game relates to a change in feel-good brain substances called neurotransmitters, particularly dopamine. (This also explains why your kid cannot put down their 3DS.) Studies using the psychology of gameplay to help people feel better physically and mentally can be found by going to Google—and there are many of them, with such good information. Let's use that information to our advantage so we can move toward answering your critical questions:

- Why am I feeling so terrible? Do I have a critical illness?
- What do I need to do to feel better?
- How can I motivate myself to continue to do the things that help me feel good?

Are you with me? Let's do this thing.

Chapter 1

Why Do I Feel Bad When My Doctor Says I'm Fine?

There Is an Answer

If one hundred thousand people end up reading this book, there will be one hundred thousand different answers; each answer is specific to each individual's body. Take heart, however: it is possible to find *your* answer. There are certain foods that commonly cause reactions, and each of us requires our own personal prescription. The interesting thing is that we can actually discover this for ourselves, and a trip to the doctor is not always required. How our bodies feel, our mind thinks, and our stomach growls is dependent on a complex algorithm that we don't even need to figure out right now. We can instead focus on broad, basic truths about what feels good and what feels bad, and how to emphasize the former.

When you break it down, the road to feeling good definitely involves taking a hard look at what you're eating and how it makes you feel. When we take in food, it's like it goes into the black box—a lot of gears, bells, and whistles. The bacteria who inhabit your gut, how well your gut pushes the food along (or doesn't!), whether or not you have the proper digestive enzymes... so many variables contributing to the end result! Once food gets into your intestine, your bacteria—some friendly, some not so friendly—use what you sent down as food, and react to it. There are trillions of bacteria in your intestines (hopefully most of them are in your large intestine where they belong and not in your small intestine). Before you personally see the benefits of the food you eat, you send a meal down to all your bacteria. Those little guys actually make vitamins for you, break down food substances, communicate with your immune system and your endocrine system—in fact, some people think of the microbiome as another body organ! Who lives down there and what they do with the cheeseburger you ate affects how you feel. According to the human microbiome project, we have around 500 to 1000 different strains of bacteria living in our gut. Some of these can make us feel bad when they thrive because of the "goo" they put out. Others are helpful and necessary. The microbiome is one seriously hot topic, and more information comes out every day.

So you have the bacteria in your gut, and then you have your cells that are lining your gut. In order for you to get all your nutrients in, and keep the bad stuff out, the gut lining has to be healthy. It would make sense that this is affected by how happy the bacteria living right next to it are. Good neighbors are so important these days! The bacteria actually make food that feeds the cells lining your gut. You see? Symbiosis. Say, for instance, you have an imbalance down there, you have some bad bacterial dudes making a bunch of inflammatory stuff. (Very precise medical terminology here.) If this leads to a breakdown in the strong structure of your gut wall lining, things are going get through that you don't want. This affects how you feel.

The next system important in how you feel relative to what you're putting in your body is your immune system. This fantastic surveillance protects you against invaders. Sixty percent of your immune system lies directly on the other side of your gut lining, just hoping to catch an invader trying to sneak in. Immune system cells are like sentries trying to keep out things that will make you sick, substances that do not belong in your body. If you have breaks in your gut wall and proteins come across that resemble part of your body—say, a protein in your joint capsule—you can actually have a reaction to *yourself*. This is called molecular mimicry and is a factor that can feed autoimmunity. When substances that shouldn't be passing the gut lining continually seep in, your immune system starts to set off a constant alarm. Constant alarm state… not good, and another reason a person can feel bad. This could be happening even if you're not having classic "stomach troubles."

Because you are dealing with a unique situation, figuring out what agrees with your body and what doesn't will require an experiment starring you. It's not a forever thing. You can do it. More about that later!

Food Sensitivities

Food sensitivities occur when our body—generally our immune system—creates a negative response to a certain food. This is different than a true "food allergy," in which a person make specific IgE antibodies to the food. With food sensitivities, the body creates a more general negative response. Luckily, these negative reactions can improve after a person's gut becomes healthier. Above, I described a situation where the gut lining has areas that "leak" (this is generally between the cells at the areas called tight junctions) and proteins squeeze through that wouldn't ordinarily be able to pass, creating inflammation. A person with this condition, commonly called "leaky gut," may not feel anything right after eating an offending food. It can take up to five days for someone to show a negative reaction. The reaction could be something really subtle like foggy thinking, or it could be something pronounced and immediate—like explosive diarrhea! (I hate it when that happens.) Figuring out what you might be sensitive to and your unique biological milieu will be part of helping you feel better.

Lifestyle Influences

What we eat, drink, do, and think throughout the day falls like snowflakes, raindrops, hail, and sunshine onto the landscape of our genetics (*and* our microbiomes), making that landscape into The Shire or... Mordor. A lot of little things add up. Good news: with so many influences, many targets for improvement pop up on the shooting range. It's all about pushing the system slowly and consistently in the direction you want to go. Throughout this program, we take small steps, keeping the eyes on the prize of vibrant, engaged, feeling-good You.

Increasing the Good

Oversimplified? Maybe. True? Definitely. There are basic things we humans need.

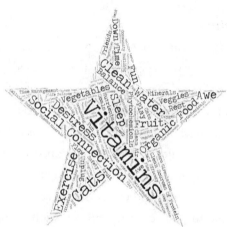

In order for our bodies and minds to function optimally, we need to pay attention to whether or not we are giving ourselves what we need. What I would like to do is to help you to identify the things you need to boost in order to obtain balance and get yourself into wonderful working order.

Booting the Bad

I could write a whole bunch about this or I could just show you a picture:

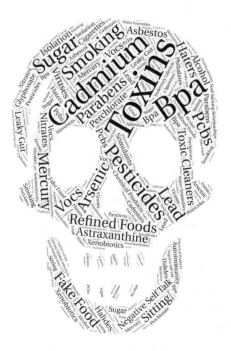

Let's find out what's leading you to feel crummy, and help you eliminate the negative.

Chapter 2

A Fresh Perspective

Harold

I want to tell you a little story about a big blue alien named Harold. Harold lived on a beautiful planet with a purple sky where everyone loved to play games. The planet's culture was built around curiosity and the quest for personal growth. He was such an amazing star on his home planet that he won the coveted top prize: an all-expenses-paid trip to the ultimate complete immersion game. He packed his bags and had a big sendoff.

In order to be immersed into the game, one had to be put to sleep, like you do before you have surgery. This seemed a little frightening to Harold, but he knew it would be worth it in the end. He had played some complex virtual-reality games that required sedation in order to use the hardware, and he trusted those with whom he was working. Besides, there were testimonials from others who had played this game who thought it was the most stunning experience of their lives.

He was brought to a majestic room full of plants and with a crystal-clear ceiling so you could see the purple sky. Reclining luxuriously onto plush pillows on a lavishly comfortable bed, singers and dancers surrounding him, he enjoyed the spectacular show as a huge crowd gathered around him to wish him well in his adventure. On a gilded table in the center of the room stood a beautiful, ominous, black onyx cup filled with crimson liquid, from which a single tendril of swirling steam snaked its way skyward. Abruptly, there came a moment like lightning. Voices hushed; the music and the chatter were cut by the knife of a screaming silence. All eyes fixed on a shaft of light falling on the cup. Time to play. He wondered if he should be frightened when he raised the vessel to his lips that would initiate the game sequence. There were no instructions for this game; he knew he would have to figure it out as he played.

The next thing he knew, he had traveled through a cramped, dark tunnel and found himself looking up at shadows of unfamiliar creatures. They were huge, many times his size, and they had him in some sort of see-through cage. There he lay, unable to sit or even pick up his head to look down at the rest of himself. A little frightened and quite hungry, he considered the challenge, "How do I get what I need?"

The basic survival game—yes, he had done this before. He needed food, shelter, tools. He decided to try and experiment with his body, but found moving it practically impossible. Concerning. He could turn his head from side to side and was able to shift around his appendages a little bit, but was limited to basically worthless wiggles. Why would the game makers create an avatar that could not do anything? He felt the tension mounting in the game, as no obvious tools seemed within his reach.

He started to panic a little bit. What if he needed to protect himself against these creatures? He noticed his breath was coming a little faster.... Now he was starting to feel ever so slightly frantic.... What if he couldn't figure out this game?

Anger! This game seemed less sophisticated than any he had played. Why didn't they give him any sort of preparation? Harold took a huge breath and all the frustration inside him came roaring out; boy, did he scream! The creatures around him started to move. Their shadows looked ominous, but he didn't want them to go away. This was a game, after all; they could be potential allies. So how could he get them to do what he needed? Limited by his inability to drive the body, he had to figure out how to communicate with them.

Cold. Unfamiliar sights, sounds. Trapped in a strange world in a body he was unable to move or even see. Someone was reaching down and picking him up. The next thing he knew, a huge soft globe the size of his head was smashed up against his face. He wondered if they were trying to smother him, but then he recognized that part of this globe had some food coming out of it. Ah, the first good thing. Later he remembered that the screaming had led to food, and he tried it again. It worked! The first tool and power boost of the game! Yes! He could tell his avatar was gaining strength. He had the scream. Scream brings warmth and globe of food. He also noticed when he kicked his appendages repetitively and tightened the muscles on the sides of his face that the creatures around him seemed more responsive. Second power boost of the game! Schweet!

When Harold entered the game, he had no idea how long he would be staying. But the longer he was there, the better he could see, and he became used to the creatures around him. He picked up new tools to meet his needs. With time, he was able to drive the body more effectively, to make it sit, then stand up and walk around. He began to be able to reproduce the sounds that he heard. Sometimes he would make a sound, and the creatures would get so excited that he made it again. Voilà—power up! It occurred to him that these creatures were probably other players in the game who were further along, and interestingly, just being with them took his score up.

As his avatar grew stronger and more adept, tools came faster. Communication with the other entities in the game began to flow and tools were exchanged between the players. Fortunately, more experienced players seemed eager to share their knowledge with younger players. New players, who entered the game completely helpless, found themselves grouped with older allies to help them survive the game and develop basic game skills at the beginning. Helping others power up and gain skills catapulted your daily score and could keep a player consistently on the leaderboard.

While the quests were not laid out as clearly as he would have liked, learning how to properly maintain and drive the avatar was rewarding in and of itself.

Interestingly, the main point of the game seemed to be pure enjoyment of the experience. He saw players leveling up, but he wasn't sure they were even aware of it. His vast experience in playing games made the structure easier to figure out. Avatar care came first. You had to give your avatar the right kind of fuel for it to function well and for you to feel well inside of it. This could be tricky, because booby traps that tapped into the avatar's pleasure system were placed in substances like artificial fuel and beverages. Another fascinating aspect of this game was that in order for his avatar to function well, he had to feel that he was in a safe place, and being with allies brought increased power and points.

Time passed, and his avatar shell grew bigger. He collected more tools and hacks, recognizing in retrospect that sometimes there were decoys. They gave the appearances of improving his game experience—that is, they seemed to bring enjoyment, but they actually sucked away his power. Most showed up in the form of pseudo-food and drink; later, they appeared as communication and strategy hacks that really seemed to work at first, then backfired.

Never before had he been in a game with such intricacies, where so many facets of one quest affected another quest. The complexity was deeply enjoyable; it was amazing when a big "aha" moment came, allowing him to recognize an initially clever pattern or strategy that was truly a trap and blast it to oblivion. Discovering new allies helped him recognize that he had been duped by certain tools and misled by other players who thought they were giving him helpful hints about the game, when in fact they were opening the door to dead-end corridors that got narrower and darker as his avatar proceeded.

One of Harold's first challenges was a prolonged survival series. His gaming group of origin was always warring with each other. Sometimes they were so kind, and other times, without any compelling provocation, they would scream and yell, creating interesting puzzles for him. How to manage and maintain his avatar in an environment where others did not understand how to manage their avatars?

At first, he tried his gaming group's suggested tools and strategies to change his avatar's state of being. He noted the change in function: slowed reflexes, more muddled thinking, a lot of fatigue, less focus on the game, and a decreased ability to remember the fact that this was actually a game, as opposed to happening directly to him. In fact, he believed that the longer an entity played this game, the more the line between game and self-blurred. That would explain the persistent use of the decoy substances that actually prevented players from leveling up and kept them from enjoying the game. These decoys obviously affected the avatar with some feedback circuitry that led to the driver repeating the behavior.

For the first seventeen years of his immersion experience ("years," unknown on Harold's planet, appeared to be the measure of how time flowed in this game), he learned a lot from his gaming group. They taught him how to use the screaming to get what he wanted, and this worked with most player/avatar duos. He learned a technique called "thought concealment" from his primary mentor, code word "Mom." This strategy used a technique to identify who knew you and truly loved you by withholding what you actually felt or thought to see if the other avatar/player could identify and act appropriately in response. Later in the game, he used this challenge with another player and they basically stopped interacting in the game with him at all! So confusing. What he thought to be an effective tool to identify those players with whom he had the closest connection—not! He leveled up when he realized that it was one of those game skills that actually took you in the wrong direction!

When Harold's avatar turned 21, he and his avatar thought they had it all figured out. Having overcome many difficult situations while growing to full size, Harold began to feel that he really was in control and taking good care of his avatar. Other players called his avatar Susan, and he deeply enjoyed working with her. They were going to be marrying someone named Tim. They were eating right, they were exercising, they were filling their body with peak moments. The joy within the machine was almost overwhelming. He saved the best moments so that they could relive them later. He had a large catalog of memory tapes that he knew would come in handy. He noted that sometimes Susan would put in memory tapes from some of their worst experiences, and he couldn't control it! It drove him crazy. Why did she keep wanting to go back to those difficult, horrible experiences?

As he considered this question, Harold realized that generally the avatar has an underlying system wired for protection, and basic needs had to be met for optimal function. He figured these things out from the very beginning, when his avatar was just a tiny creature. It was absolutely essential to be around other supportive players, to feel safe, to feel like you're moving forward in the game and having success, to feel like you're able to take care of yourself, and to feel that you are in a fair and just place both for yourself and others. The best environment was a state of flow, with interesting challenges to keep leveling up in the game. Clues and quests appeared in the form of little brain stumpers during those times he found it difficult to control his avatar's actions. It was a signal from the unit, a code for a primal need that was necessary for optimal avatar functioning.

So, re-living troubling memories… what could the purpose be in terms of basic needs? He noticed that these memories generally left Susan with a strong emotion: sadness, anger, desire for fairness, need for resolution. Interesting puzzle. Within those past experiences that Susan kept living over and over again in her head, Harold noticed that a messaging function regarding one of these critical elements was malfunctioning. Harold brought up some of the repetitive videos when the other player called "Mom" would have a communication breakdown and misfire, ignoring, speaking down, or yelling at his avatar. This kind of experience led to a reflexive flurry of messages in his command central—all negative—and mystifyingly about Susan herself instead of the malfunctioning unit "Mom."

Another thing he noticed, on those days when Susan played a lot of these old negative tapes, was that he had less control over her. At the end of the day when he took a survey of all systems, he found that the happiness meter shifted toward the negative when a lot of those old tapes had been run. Old negative memories led to feeling bad in the now.

What if there were a way to play current videos to get Susan to stay in her present (which was currently wonderful) and to start to play more fun future videos? It would be like pouring fresh water into a glass of dirty water, slowly displacing the old with the new. He couldn't wait to try his new idea. He called his strategy, "The real now and bright future plan."

"The next time she starts to put in one of those old tapes, I am going to grab it and put in a good tape!" thought Harold. He tried this with marginal results; Susan overrode him and kept putting in the old tapes. What if he could identify and address the need that went along with the strong emotions she conjured up each time she played the familiar negative reels? Maybe he could put in a tape that was specific for that. Hmmm….

He could tell he was onto something here. There was one tape in particular that she continually replayed; he learned to recognize the emotion of sadness and the feeling of inadequacy that came along with it. Even though his avatar had done a lot of amazing things! Up to this point in the game, this one memory could squash *all* of those good memories. Conquering this challenge could certainly level him up if he could figure it out.

He grabbed several of the best memories he could find, ones where his avatar was clearly showing her strong points, making the grade, showing her ability to achieve, and feeling super happy. Somehow, Susan had stored these on the bottom shelf. The next time one of those tapes started to move toward the player, he was ready. Right after his avatar watched the old "standard" and went to that negative place, he started to put in tapes with better memories. There was the one when she graduated from high school, there was the one when she did something kind for a friend, and there was another one of a fantastic vacation when she was actually getting along with the avatar called "Mom." The first time he tried it—no change. But when he started to do this every time those old tapes showed up, the happiness meter stopped dipping so low. At the end of the day, his instrument surveys showed an improvement in the overall mood level. Boom! Power up!

It seemed like he and Susan were starting to work in concert. Clearly they both had some degree of control over what kind of game they were playing. He could not always override Susan's impulses, but he learned to expect that. There were surprises; Susan had a baby, a peak moment that was definitely going to join the good tapes on the top shelf of the video catalog. After the baby, though, his avatar didn't seem to run as smoothly; balance was off, there was some extra mass involved. Harold focused on trying to control the kind of fuel that was coming in, but this proved difficult, because he and his avatar were working on developing the new player—the baby—and this led to erratic schedules and even more erratic fuel consumption. He and Susan stayed in one gaming area instead of going to a "job." He looked to identify behaviors that would bring pleasure, which by now he knew without question was a player's prime objective.

For boosting overall mood, certain foods seemed to fit the bill. However the more they relied on those foods, the less efficiently his avatar seemed to function. Another trap! Back to basics: avatar care and handling, and the ongoing question of what the avatar's basic and changing needs seemed to be. Harold noted that the only significant change, besides the addition of the new player onto their gaming team, was Susan leaving her job. Could this be a message of boredom to central communication from the avatar's executive functioning unit? Perhaps the eating behavior was more about lack of challenge instead of hunger. He made a plan to identify what "hungry" felt like, so he could send signals to Susan that would help her eat when she was hungry and do something interesting when she was bored.

In command central, one of the most enjoyable parts of his day was actually when he got to engage in battle: overcoming obstacles and truly playing! It was clear that each avatar had their own personal menu of chosen challenges, almost as though perfectly selected for each being. The player running the show had to first identify these obstacles, and then figure out how to get their avatar to overcome them. It seemed clear from a young age that his avatar was drawn to a certain kind of fuel that led to inefficient function. Initially, this fuel was always in a colorful package that Susan had an immediate reaction to as soon as it came within her line of vision. He could feel the changes within his avatar just at the sight of this fuel. Over the years, it became clear that after she consumed this fuel, command central would not work as well and there would be a drive for rest, as in, "I have to lie down right now." It seemed clear that the built-in, rudimentary neural network protection system did not identify this as a negative influence. How could he take his avatar from craving and loving something that was hurting her to a state of indifference toward the item, especially when there seemed to be a bodily urge built into the booby trap? Harold liked to work backwards with these kinds of problems. He started with the solution: his avatar would only rarely use the fuel that caused the malfunction. How could he craft this battle? He starting by naming the enemy. Susan called them sweets. He gave this fuel a new name that more aptly identified its treacherous nature: Señor Sweet and Vicious! Game on!

He made a list—a game plan of action steps he planned to take his avatar through—with the goal of Susan losing her cravings for Señor Sweet and Vicious and rendering him Señor Sweet Indifference. He saw things unfolding like this:

- Susan keeps a journal of her food and the way she is feeling
- Susan recognizes that sweets make her feel bad, tired, and foggy after she eats them
- Susan decides she wants to feel better
- Susan identifies the triggers that lead her to eat the sweets
- Susan modifies her environment so that the physical triggers are gone
- Susan makes a plan for when she gets triggered and writes it down
- Susan identifies the reward or underlying emotional need that is filled when she eats treats

- Susan identifies other ways to fulfill her need besides the treats and includes them in her strategies
- Susan practices her plan in her head every morning, seeing herself make good choices
- Susan finds a group of other people who are also trying to do the same thing for support
- Susan uses a game approach to go without treats for a week
- Susan sees that she can control this behavior and feels encouraged
- Susan's craving for sweets is reduced, but not entirely gone
- Susan identifies the healthiest options that she can use when she makes the decision to have a treat
- Susan talks with her healthcare provider about why she might be craving sweets and learns about insulin levels
- Susan works with her body, using food combinations to decrease the drive for sweets and avoid high insulin levels
- Susan maintains this style of eating for a month
- Susan loses her craving for sweets

He started to watch the other avatars that leveled up quickly, trying to figure out what they were doing. He noticed that they spent significant time in introspection. What if during that time they were able to connect with their avatar driver? What if he could somehow contact Susan? Maybe if they intentionally worked together, they could level up faster. He had seen other players take quiet breaks. What did they call that? Meditation? Prayer? Reflection? Yeah, that's right. What a great idea. He was going to try and reach her.

The next day when they woke up, he directed her to get into a comfortable position and take slow, deep breaths. He used the joystick control in command central to move her hand to pick up her headphones and put them on, connecting them to her iPhone. She searched for binaural beats on YouTube and started to play them while she took slow, deep breaths. He took breaths at the same time, starting to feel a deep sense of calm and expansion. It was as though their minds began to meld. He had a better understanding of her impulses, and she seemed to recognize that she had an extra source of power and control. They worked out together, getting into a routine. They would start with connecting through relaxation and breathing, and then they would link up through simple body movements where he controlled the movement of her hands and she let him control her—total symbiosis. After that, she let him put in all the great tapes that they loved. They would relive the stunning moments in her history when she felt amazing. Then they would visit their future—all the dreams, the visions, the plans—and they would live *in* them for a few moments every day. Harold picked challenges that he turned into quests, imagining the battles, making a plan for how he would level up, knowing that honoring the basic needs of the avatar invariably led to more points.

Then, one day, something happened and Susan lost interest and focus. She seemed tired. Harold wondered how he could lift her up. Then he realized—duh!—that he had to *let her in* on the game. Up to this point, he had been creating their objectives on his own. He realized that avatars enjoy games as much as players; this could be the key to getting Susan fired up about collaborating with him. Life's the game, after all.

What If...?

What if your body was your avatar shell and it was all a big game?

In your life game, have you ever felt misled by other "players," or bought into some slick tools that have turned out to be taking you in the wrong direction? What if the little person in the machine was you, and each little choice on which arm to lift, which way to look, and which food to choose was coming from a control room (not unlike the control room in the popular animated film, *Inside Out*)? What if that tiny mini-me was imbued with all your best traits, best judgments, and even qualities that you want to possess but don't feel as though you yet fully grasp? What if you joined forces and started questing together to bring yourself a vibrant, fulfilled life of health and joy?

What if it became fun to make the right choice? Can we please get some dopamine in the control room?! How could you score a dopamine surge for *not* having a decadent dark chocolate mudslide cake? Easy: when not having it becomes part of winning the game of you. Whether you know it or not, a lot of your choices are directed by a physical urge to create more feel-good chemicals in your body. Research shows that these feel-good chemicals can actually come from playing games, and this knowledge can help you change your behavior.

Are you the avatar or are you the player? Perhaps you already feel a connection to the little voice in your head. The Feel Good Again program is about connecting with our own Harold while using fun little hacks and games to power up our lives, incorporating functional medicine principles, high-tailing it into feeling good, and hitting our stride. You can feel better, and this book can show you how. As we set out to engage in our personal game of life, we, like Harold, have to take stock of where we are in the moment. I expect nothing less than a massive health revolution for you, but before that happens, a little prep work must be done. Time to craft your personal medical transformation.

Ever tried to come up with a story off the top of your head? Hard. The beginning is critical, especially understanding the main character: their motivation, joys, sorrows, and quirks. And then there's setting the scene: recent victories, tragedies or painful histories... maybe they just landed upside down in a squishy pink baby's body with no clue like our pal Harold!

The first thing Harold did was take stock. What do we have here? Where are we? What are our assets? Liabilities? Alrighty, since you are the star of this medical transformation adventure, let's focus on you and your story. What is your current state of physical and emotional health? What past experiences affect your future? Any habits you plan to shift? Looking for the underlying root cause of your symptoms? Let's pin down our point of entry into the maze.

Before we can make *your* amazing game, though, you need some instruction. Why didn't Harold get any instructions when he was plopped into the baby's body? Because part of his game was figuring it out. Fortunately, some avatar driver out there decided they should make this information public, and you get all the benefit! Here we go!

Chapter 3

Your Avatar Driver's Manual

Congratulations on your choice of personal avatar! Your avatar is a precision instrument designed to provide many years of pleasurable engagement and gaming. Life is a virtual-reality sandbox with no set rules, in which the quests are set by you, and are specific to your environment and personal growth needs. Default mode of play is determined by the arrangement of your personal environment; most players choose a mix of survival and creative mode, although for many, this is an unconscious choice. This guide will help you achieve optimum performance by explaining how you can adjust your avatar's system through provision of basic needs and fuel. Read the instructions carefully for best results with your product!

Instructions for Care

Fuel:

Each avatar comes complete with its own unique set of fuel needs, in addition to an accessory system of co-inhabitants that live on top of and within the avatar itself. There are basic rules which can help the player identify optimal fuel, and these include:

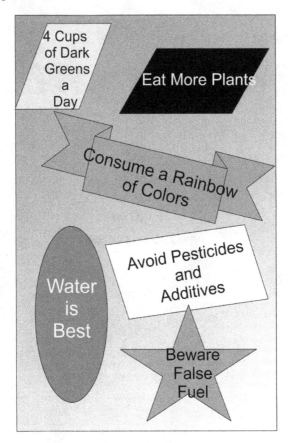

Bonus Features

Your avatar may come equipped with a special adventure feature that elicits a response to one or more mystery substances! If you are so lucky to have received an avatar with this feature, congratulations! Part of your quest will be unlocking the key to identifying your mystery substance! These mystery substances trigger special reactions when they are ingested: sometimes bloating, sometimes abdominal pain, sometimes nasal congestion, joint pain, fatigue, muscle aches, or rashes. This special feature is a bonus provided at no extra charge!

Basic Needs for Avatar Executive Function

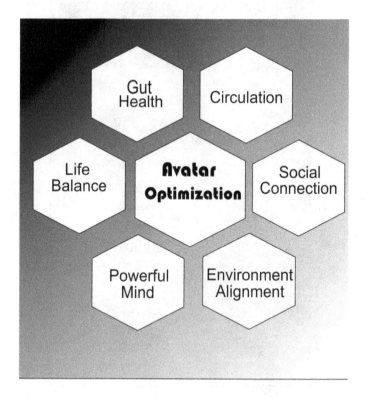

Basic Needs for Avatar Physical Performance

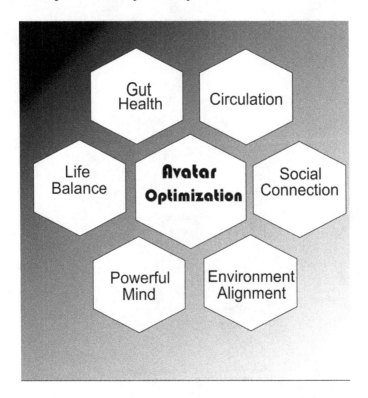

Game Rules

Objective:

The objective of the game is to guide your avatar through quests that will lead to leveling up through the Game Level Pyramid while maximizing enjoyment and connection. One initial goal is to make direct contact with the executive functioning system of your avatar so that you may work in tandem. When you achieve this, you will level up faster and accumulate points more quickly. The point value of enjoying the game cannot be overestimated!

Self Actualization: achieving one's full potential, morality, creativity, problem-solving

Meeting Self Esteem Needs: confidence, achievement, success, respect

Meeting Relationship Needs: friends, intimate relationships, and social network, family

Meeting Safety Needs: security of body, employment, resources, family, health, and property

Meeting physiological needs: food, water, warmth, rest, biotransformation, circulation

Important points to remember during the game:

- As you go through quests, the more happiness, pleasure and enjoyment that you create for your avatar without damaging the unit, while simultaneously avoiding booby-traps, the more additional power to the system, points, and progress up the Game Level Pyramid.

- Your avatar adapts to physiologically resemble the five other player/avatar duos with whom you spend the most time. Choose your allies wisely.
- Proper group play will take the whole group up the Game Level Pyramid faster.
- Your avatar is fully equipped to complete all necessary missions for achievement of the final objective. You as the player must unlock these competencies.
- Extra points are given to the players who extend the most assistance to others throughout the length of their game.

Good Luck!
And May the Odds Be Ever in Your Favor!

Welcome, Newly Awakened Avatar Driver!

This could be a little bit of a shock to your system; don't you worry, it will be okay. I know you're saying to yourself, "How could I have missed this!?" The fact is, many avatar drivers go their entire lives without realizing that they are playing the ultimate game. Fantastic for you, this awakening! And more great news: you have a few more tools than Harold did when he started his quest, and it's likely that you have already covered some of these first steps with your healthcare provider. Think of this as a checkpoint, like pulling your Ferrari into the pit for a little lookie-under-the-hoodie. Getting a baseline and ruling out life-threatening illness in your avatar with a basic checkup and conventional lab work is a great first step. Typical labs to help rule out immediate life-threatening issues would include:

- Complete Blood Count (CBC) that will look for infections and abnormalities of the blood such as anemia and blood cancers.

- Urinalysis to identify any glucose in the urine, which can suggest diabetes. Protein in the urine can let us know if there's some problem or infection in your body's filtration system.
- Comprehensive metabolic panel evaluates the blood's electrolyte balance along with kidney and liver function.
- TSH and free T4 are typically ordered by conventional physicians as part of a panel evaluating fatigue and multiple symptom issues.
- Basic preventive screening as recommended by a health provider that you trust shares your perspective on medical intervention.

Perhaps you've already had this sort of evaluation from your provider and everything has been normal, like Carol and Chase. (And I bet your provider didn't even mention the fact that you're in the middle of a big virtual reality game!) If you are in that space in which how you're feeling doesn't match what your labs show, then the next step toward understanding what is holding your avatar back in terms of health and wellness could be going to see a functional medicine provider. They would ask a *whole lot* of questions to get to know you, and probably order further testing which could include:

1. **Nutritional evaluation** that looks at how well you are processing nutrients and the adequacy of vitamins and minerals. Functional medicine providers (some of whom are MDs, naturopaths, chiropractors, nutritionists, nurse practitioners, traditional Chinese medicine practitioners, etc.) are familiar with nutritional evaluations if your doctor is uncomfortable ordering this kind of lab work.

2. **Complete stool testing** that will show how well your body is mechanically processing food and give insight into inflammation and any possible infections that you may harbor

in your intestine. It will also help determine whether you may have imbalances in your microbiota. Your microbiota is all the bacteria that live in and around you. Turns out that these guys are critical for proper functioning and minimization of symptoms. They talk to our nervous system and our immune system and are critical to maintaining a happy body.

3. **Evaluation of hormonal levels** and a complete thyroid panel which can uncover hidden hypothyroidism, not always identified by just checking TSH and free T4. Checking hormone levels can be helpful in some cases, depending on the symptoms. Often I focus on the gastrointestinal system, reducing stress and addressing lifestyle issues at first, and seeing how far that takes a person in feeling better before considering further hormone level testing.

4. **Markers for inflammation, cytokines, and autoantibodies.** These labs help identify and quantify inflammation and autoimmunity, and are sometimes ordered initially with basic lab work, depending on what symptoms you bring to your provider. Tracking to monitor response such as a decline in inflammation requires initial tests to see how things change. Work in conjunction with your physician to see if any tests to evaluate your system for autoimmune problems are appropriate.

5. **Genetics evaluation,** including single nucleotide polymorphisms (SNPs.) SNPs are tiny variations in our genetic code that can affect lots of processes in our body. Some change the effectiveness of enzymes, some affect transporters that we need in our cells, and many have been identified as possible targets for improvement through nutritional supplementation. It's about looking for these small differences whose expression could be influenced by simple means like eating more broccoli!

Regarding genetic testing: using genetic data holds some controversy, and has been hotly debated. The fact is, people will be using these services and bringing them to their doctor with a big question mark on their faces; patients will drive the need for physicians to take the time to understand and use the data responsibly, no matter what I write. The medical community is going to have to put on their BGPs and BBPs and figure it out. 23andMe is an online lab that gives your whole genome for about $200. Some clients express concern that they don't want anyone else having or using their genetic data, and in that case, simply use an alternate name to protect your privacy.

When the raw genetic data is received, it can be evaluated using various computer programs or apps that will identify SNPs whose influence can be altered by nutrition or supplements. When we are talking genetics, the words get long, boring, and oh-so-complex. Unless you have a lot of spare time and brain power, find someone to guide you through the process. It can really yield useful information. Just today I reviewed a client's genetics with her, and it turned out she had variations that gave us some stellar treatment targets that involved simple vitamins! I've included some resources in the appendix for working with your own raw genetic data. Check it out if you're feeling brave!

Status Questionnaires

I like to use several questionnaires to identify current avatar/driver state. The links to these can be found on my website at www.sunnygmd.com or in the appendix at the back of this book. They address the physical and emotional. Having a baseline allows us to measure change. Evolution in our health tends to be gradual, and many times when we're in the thick of things, we are unable to recognize that things are changing unless we are taking snapshots in time.

- Feel Good Again Questionnaire: www.sunnygmd.com
- For those with anxiety: www.thecalculator.co/health/ Generalized-Anxiety-Disorder-GAD-7-Calculator-802.html
- For those with depressive symptoms, the blues, or lack of get up and go: www.mdcalc.com/phq-9-patient-health-questionnaire-9/
- Values in Action Questionnaire: http://www.viacharacter.org/ www/Character-Strengths-Survey

⟶ *Assignment* ⟶

Stop everything you're doing right now, go to my website, and take these questionnaires. The Feel Good Again questionnaire is all about where you are right now. If you have anxiety or depressive symptoms, I recommend you include the GAD 7 and the PHQ 9. The Values in Action Questionnaire will help you understand your strongest points for effectively driving your avatar and reinforcing your superpowers.

Supplementation and Nutrition

For best function, your avatar requires specific nutrients. Acquiring them used to be as simple as eating a balanced diet. Unfortunately, over the past 20 to 30 years, our food pool has really changed. It's a little harder to get all the nutrients we need through safe food sources, so I suggest several supplements for everybody across the board. One is a good multivitamin that's manufactured by a company that is Good Manufacturing Practice (GMP)-certified and represents products that are produced and controlled according to quality standards.

- Multivitamin/multi-mineral supplement.
- Vitamin D3, 1000 international units daily. Levels need to be checked to determine that you're not getting too much or

too little. Work with your provider to get your levels within recommended range. See the appendix for optimal values.

- Omega-3 fatty acids or a fish oil/ krill oil supplement. I recommend 2000 mg for the average person. Those with inflammatory and auto-immune issues may benefit from a higher dose; talk to your healthcare provider about dosing recommendations.
- B complex vitamin daily.
- Daily probiotic, 25 Billion CFUs or fermented foods (like kombucha, sauerkraut, pickled veggies, kimchi) every day.

Solid recommendations include eating an organic, whole food diet—that means as near to the original form as possible. The idea of avoiding GMO foods seems to hold merit, if you're reading the research. Wondering why organic? Considering that you are a big cloud of microorganisms of which you just happen to be the largest, taking care of that lovely cloud should be at the top of your personal agenda. Avoiding pesticides on produce is a way to help manage the microbes living in your gut. When you eat it, they eat it. The Environmental Working Group puts out great guides in terms of which fruits and vegetables contain the most pesticides, and therefore should always be eaten in organic form if possible. See the appendix for current recommended supplements and more information on the "Dirty Dozen" and the "Clean 15."

Eat the rainbow; see if you can get all the colors in every day. No argument from anyone about that. Moreover, different people need different styles of eating for optimal health. We are all trying to find the Holy Grail in terms of diet, and it is just not there. We're snowflakes, right? We have our own genetics, our own little set of bacteria that live in us, and our own exposure history and ability to detox from our exposures. This leads to one size does *not* fit all; thus the personal avatar adventure.

The Mirror

Knowing oneself at a precise moment opens the possibility for personal reinvention.

We've covered the basics of use and care for your gaming unit. At this point in your experience, you have acquired tools and strategies, many of which are necessary and excellent. The following section will assist you in analyzing your current operating system as well as exploring possibilities for an upgrade.

For several years, I lived in a house with few mirrors. I didn't even really think about it until we moved to a new house and suddenly I was looking at myself in the mirror every day while brushing my teeth. Of course I started to scrutinize, because that's what we do when we stare into a mirror, noticing how things have changed.

Lots of us brush our teeth, staring at a mirror, but as you engage in your new game, "mirror gazing" will be a key strategy to help you figure out how to level up. We want to capture a snapshot of you and all your habits, thoughts, quirks, strong points, and glorious flaws. We started with questionnaires, now on with some journaling. Time to make a list—a big list. Most of us can only do this for a short period of time (it's kind of tedious to put every little thing on paper or on your phone). But now is that time. The goal is to obtain a complete picture of you in this moment.

You've seen shots in movies that initially just look like an abstract graphic image until the camera zooms in and you realize that the picture is made up of many little pixels that are actually pictures, right? If we zoom in on ourselves, we find that we are created of pixelated habits: habits of thought, self-talk, food choice, emotions, actions.... You get where I'm going. Let's consider it this way: imagine you are like Harold, the big blue alien who entered the game as a baby with a blank playing field. Close your eyes and imagine for a moment a tiny you sitting at a control panel in your head and pushing a lever forward to lift your arm. Now the other arm. Imagine your tiny self talking into a microphone in your head, making the connection as the words come out of your mouth. Drive that avatar, baby! Walk your avatar around the room. This slight perceptive shift can completely change your ability to control your actions, thoughts, and habits.

Over your lifetime, you have gathered useful tools, created strategies, strengthened your avatar with booster power, possibly been bamboozled by instant gratification, or duped into walking down narrowing corridors by false allies or well-intended players who really didn't know the rules of the game. Look back in your life and see if you can identify some behaviors that seemed to work well for you initially, and now are actually taking you in the wrong direction in your life and health.

Maybe you've been given medications to cover up symptoms instead of trying to identify why the symptoms are there in the first place. Perhaps you have some comfort or distraction habits, such as eating to fill an empty space, or watching television to escape stress. These may work in the short term, but over the longer haul can lead folks to a dead end and a shorter life. All of us receive well-meaning advice from family and friends, healthcare providers, but let's be honest: at this point, those things have not worked, right? It is time to back up, do a little rewind, and rethink our old strategies. Everything we do is habitual and changeable. Your first job is simply to identify all those pixels, habitual thoughts, and actions. No judgment. We're just trying to figure out where you are. Later on, you will tease out which ones are taking you further in the game—leading to health, fulfillment, energy, happiness, peace, love—and which ones are pulling you down and dropping your score, taking you to dead ends and decreasing your power.

—⁓⁓ *Assignment* —⁓⁓

For the next two to three days, you are going to record everything. This can be in a virtual form, such as using your notes app on your phone. I find I capture the most if I use the voice recorder option on my phone and put it into a note that I can email to myself. The form doesn't matter. A spiral-bound notebook works just fine. Journaling and self-reflection is not always easy, and many people need little reminders throughout the day to remember to write things down. I suggest setting an alarm on your phone or on your watch that will simply bring you back to the task. The more information you have, the more we have to work with.

You may find yourself unable to maintain this throughout a whole day. Please don't beat yourself up. Maybe try for a few hours at a time, or even start with 15 minutes. Just get as much information as you can. Important things to note are: times when you feel good or great, activities that bring you energy, habitual negative thoughts, repetitive concerns, feelings of anxiety, thoughts or actions associated with subsequent emotions, like making a poor food choice and feeling subsequent guilt, petting the cat and a feeling of contentment or calm, or listening to music and feeling your anxiety level dropping.

As you begin this exercise, think of yourself as the little guy in your head taking inventory. This removes some of the charge around a difficult task. Give yourself a big pat on the back after you complete this journaling. Not only is it a lot of work, it is amazing to take stock and know oneself. If you have done this electronically, it might be helpful to print out your information so you can use it to create your quest.

Exercise: Visualization
Shut your eyes, and imagine rolling up your papers into a cylinder. Now I want you to picture that cylinder and start to decorate it with

your favorite colors. Make it beautiful. Give it swirls. Give it polka dots. Give it stripes! While you're imagining, I'd like you to picture all the questionnaires you did and imagine rolling them up and putting them inside the cylinder, too. Notice in your mind the air around the cylinder; it's a beautiful color. In fact, it's your favorite color, glowing with energy. Now, as you look at the cylinder in your mind, notice that it's starting to move, and now you recognize it for what it is: a caterpillar. It is the most gorgeous caterpillar you have seen in your entire life. All those experiences, habits, thoughts, emotions, and strategies, they're all rolled up and represent one gorgeous caterpillar. You. Now picture that breathtaking caterpillar in the most dazzlingly beautiful forest; watch it weave its cocoon. And we're going to time-lapse to the time when the butterfly emerges. Out of that cocoon comes a stunning butterfly whose equal has never been seen. That butterfly is you. You floating on the breeze, in and among the flowers, ferns, along a steep ocean cliff, bouncing and enjoying. Lighting on a mountainside and following a flowing river. You notice the butterfly changing. The wings begin to look more muscular, stronger. It starts to fly with purpose and intention. Feel yourself in the butterfly as it becomes a bird, soaring over a fantastic landscape, powerfully beating majestic wings to climb higher, surrounded by an air of peace and presence. Focused positive intentions and a calm mind spread, gradually filling the body with a vibrating congruence, letting you clearly see the personal possibilities that come when harnessing inner wisdom. You transform as you embrace your strengths, and the old paradigm of your life, health, limiting beliefs—those pieces of your puzzle that need to be shifted or even let go of—move to the edges of your body and become scintillating fiery magic, much cherished, and honored as a part of you, and gracefully released onto the breeze, propelling you straight up like an arrow. Welcome to the Future You.

Time Travel: Meet Future You

If you are considering an upgrade to your current model (if you're reading this, you are), now is the time to select the features you desire in your next revision. Operating systems must be gradually overwritten, as system complexity prevents a complete reboot. In order to write the code most appropriate for your avatar's development, we begin with the end in mind.

Can't drive to Vancouver without knowing you're going to Vancouver, right? Now comes the fun part: we're going to engage the creative part of your brain to craft an image of your desired future. Time to drop the limits that have been placed upon you by your physicians, by your family, by your history. Wipe 'em clean. No place for limits in this exercise!

I like a whiteboard for this exercise, because it gives you a lot of space to draw and write. Especially fun with multicolored markers! Fast-forward your personal time reel and imagine what your perfect day is like in two years, after you've been through this work. Details, details! What time do you get up? How do you feel in your body? What is your energy level? What do you think when you get up? What is the main mood that drives your day? What relationships are there, what relationships are gone? Have you discontinued medications? Activities, hobbies, social groups, work… don't hold back. Future You feels great and loves life's journey.

It may seem as though these questions are outside the realm of medicine, but *au contraire*. Your health is a whole-body experience. There are those whose body may be mechanically functioning okay from a physical perspective, but the way they *feel* in their body is limited by other factors; they lack the vibrance, energy, and mood they desire. There is no way to separate the body from the mind, so we will address it all. In fact, you may have noticed that I didn't suggest that you put in a dream weight or anything like that. This is more about focusing on how you feel, because habits that lead us toward health generally make us feel better and the physical form follows. If we focus on creating a life filled with words, deeds, and thoughts that center around wellness, health will come. Imagine your body as a cup that's filled with everything that makes you, *you*. Some of those things you love; some of those things you'd rather not have in the cup. One big technique we will use is displacement—putting more good stuff in the cup makes less room for the bad stuff.

Time Travel: Meet Future You and Questions to Consider

Future You

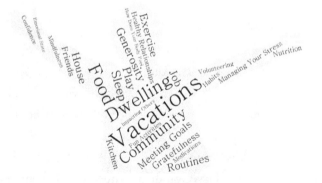

What are your possibilities? Hopes? Dreams?

—✦— *Assignment* —✦—

Capture Future You in your journal, subdividing thoughts into the realms of physical, mental, emotional, work, social. This exercise is critical as it will help you divine your quest and allow you to set tiny goals to propel you forward.

Drawing the Map, Designing the Journey

Starting point: check. Destination: check. All we have to do is fill in the middle part! There something magic about actually writing down the progression of skills, habits, and growth that will bring you to your destination. This is a quest, implying more than just a quick fix. We want to split the long journey into small chunks that are manageable. When you look at the exercise where you captured your future self, you probably see some desires that stand out. These may be symptom resolution, changes in thought processes and mood, changes in your environment, self-discipline, and all of these could be excellent places to start. Our transformation to Feel Good Again always begins with the same four steps:

- Step 1. Check In: current state (Feel Better Again Questionnaire)
- Step 2. Take Stock: of where I am today (The Mirror)
- Step 3. Time Travel: to meet my future self
- Step 4: Draw the Map: design the journey between here and there.

This is where you start to fill in the steps.

Design of a Sample Quest

Let's say that future me wants to take a daily mile long walk.

Goal: Daily Mile-Long Walk

Now I imagine, "What is the step immediately before I am taking a daily mile-long walk?"

Goal: Daily Mile-Long Walk
- Taking short walks daily and adding some long walks, several times a week
- Daily mile-long walk

Next: "What is the step immediately before I am taking short walks daily with a long walk, several times a week?" A plan is starting to take shape:

Goal: Daily Mile-Long Walk
- Taking short walks daily
- Taking short walks daily and adding some long walks, several times a week
- Daily mile-long walk.

After I write that down, I realize that there is a missing step (maybe even a few) in between "taking short walks daily with an occasional long walk" and just "taking short walks daily," and that is planning time in my schedule for longer walks. I have to put in an extra step between these as I'm planning my journey. My plan now reads:

Goal: Daily Mile-Long Walk
- Taking short walks daily
- Making time in my schedule to take an occasional long walk
- Taking short walks daily and adding some long walks, several times a week
- Making time in my schedule to take a daily long walk

As I continue to craft this quest, I can see that time is not the only issue, I also have to actually remember to do this and make it a priority.

Since I know that it is easier to fit things into your day when you plan them, this becomes part of my quest. Let's say for instance that I don't take a daily walk currently, I begin by taking an occasional walk here and there. I might structure it like this:

Goal: Daily Mile-Long Walk
- Putting a daily walk into my planner
- Setting a reminder, so I remember to take my walk
- Taking short walks daily
- Making time in my schedule to take an occasional long walk
- Taking short walks daily and adding some long walks, several times a week
- Making time in my schedule and putting a daily long walk in my planner

What if I'm not doing any walking at all right now? All we have to do is add in some steps before the above. It could look something like this:

Goal: Daily Mile-Long Walk
- Stepping out of my house daily
- Going to the mailbox daily to get the mail
- Walking an extra 10 feet away from my mailbox after I get the mail and back
- Slowly extending the distance I walk away from the mailbox
- Putting a daily walk into my planner
- Setting a reminder, so I remember to take my walk
- Taking short walks daily
- Making time in my schedule to take an occasional long walk
- Taking short walks daily with a long walk, several times a week

- Making time in my schedule and putting a daily long walk in my planner
- Daily mile-long walk

You get the idea here. Working backwards doesn't come naturally initially. It may even seem like a hassle. It is important that you take the time to do this and identify your next step—then the only thing you focus on is that next step. You don't have to worry about running the marathon. You worry about getting up out of the chair. Take your avatar wherever it may be at this moment and skooch it in the direction you want to go. Each level earns you more points and takes you further up on the Game Level Pyramid.

You may be thinking that all this is well and good, but that the idea of doing this continuously seems exhausting. I totally agree. That's why we don't do this continuously. This is a cycle. You work on movement up the Game Level Pyramid for two months at a time. At the end of each cycle, players must take time to solidify the systemic wiring they have put in place. Called stabilization, this time period allows the avatar/driver unit to maintain and reinforce the newly laid brain connections. When the driver is ready, the cycle restarts.

Step 1. **Check In: current state (Feel Good Again Questionnaire)**

Step 2. **Take Stock: of where I am today (The Mirror)**

Step 3. **Time Travel: to meet my future self**

Step 4: **Draw the Map: design the journey between here and there**

Sometimes designing this journey requires a guide, a health provider of some sort to give you the medical framework beyond the basics of eliminating foods that may actually be causing symptoms, bolstering your microbiome and gut health, diminishing toxins, and improving self-care, and that is positively fine. You may have an issue with chronic, low-lying infections that have gone unrecognized, and this requires some medical sleuthing to get to the bottom of the matter. There are as many different paths as there are people. The advantage to the cyclic approach is that you get to keep reevaluating both the goal and the plan. Nothing is perfect; nothing has to be perfect. Perfect is the enemy of the good. As imperfect people, we must plan to make mistakes and let them be our teachers.

> *"Our greatest weakness lies in giving up. The most certain way to succeed is always to try just one more time."*
> **—Thomas A. Edison**

We've taken stock, visioned our future self, and created a path. Now how are we going to make this fun? In the next chapter, we'll explore the creation of your own personal game, immersing you in imaginative play and possibility as you undergo your medical transformation.

Chapter 4

The Elements of the Game

Remember when Harold had to come up with a strategy to try and give his avatar, Susan, a boost? He countered negative tapes in her head by recognizing her positive attributes, skills, positive memories, etc. We will craft your quest using your strong points; as you grow and develop, you'll collect more skills and power-ups.

Power Boosters

Let's analyze your data. We want to organize, in a "keep versus toss" fashion, all those little details about you. Grab yourself some nice highlighters. Pick your favorite color, and mark up the positives in your notes. No judging allowed. When you're done, hopefully you have identified good things about your life right now that pump you up and personal qualities that will help you in your journey. Use the results of your Values in Action questionnaire to identify your avatar's best points.

As you continue through your medical transformation process, be on the lookout for more thoughts, activities, memories, projects, and relationships that boost your energy, bring you joy, calm you down when you are anxious, and take you to your happy place. This is your list of awesome: your Power Boosters! If there's nothing that makes you feel awesome *yet*, no problem, let's make a list of things or activities that are interesting and can draw your attention, like topics or activities you have enjoyed in the past, fantasies that can bring you joy or calm you down, or things you *would like* to take you to your most grounded and peaceful state—like the one Susan achieved when Harold played feel-good tapes for her.

⇒ \~\⁄⁓ *Assignment: Create Your Superpower Pack* ⇒ \~\⁄⁓

After you have completed the exercises above, use the information along with the results from your Values in Action questionnaire in order to make a 3 x 5 card that has your top five superpowers written on it. Make it fun, make it interesting, and make it eye-catching. This is your personal Superpower Pack! Keep it in your pocket as a reminder to use your Superpowers for good.

You can add to this list at any time, focusing on things that increase your energy, improve your mood, and calm you down when you're anxious to use as tools in your game. As you list these, you can soup them up with fun names. Playful approaches to self-care can turn the "I shoulds" into "I want tos." For instance, slow deep breathing is one of my Power Boosters, but I don't call it "slow deep breathing," I call it "Power Breath." Just saying that makes me a little happier. I'm going to my "Power Breath" now. Pardon me... Okay, I'm back.

Monsters, Mayhem and Battles—Oh My!

What fun is an adventure without some bad guys to battle? Remember Harold when he created the quest to overcome Señor Sweet and Vicious? Now it's your turn. We started by identifying the good stuff, now let's figure out what you'd like to change. Much in the same way that you listed those positives, let's make a list of things you want to do differently, habits to break, moods to soothe, and patterns to evolve. It all gives you plenty of material with which you can create your game. These become your monsters, challenges, the dastardly sneaky villains in your quest. They are critical, because they grant our superhero selves the opportunity to battle and be victorious. We will not choose to battle all of them right from the start—in fact, this game works best when you start small.

On a finer point, the more desperate you are, the more creative you ought to be with this. Humor helps, seriously. Some personal examples:

- 5 o'clock glass of wine becomes... *Marquis d'Vino*, the evil villain who lures me into drinking the poison potion that steals my self-control and leaves me irritable for the rest of the evening.
- I don't feel like exercising becomes... *Mlle. Bigger Booty*, who cackles evil laughter when I listen to her siren song and sit on the couch. (And, seriously, I actually have a sound effect that is evil laughter, which I play when we are battling.)
- My little negative voice that tells me things like "you'll never get this book done" or "your house is a wreck" becomes... *Seraphina NoGood, the Dark Angel*. As an aside, I like to sic *Magnificent Macy the White Angel* (she is my clever, mischievous fount of positivity, just like her namesake, my dog) on her—she's got my back. They have fantastic battles; Macy has been known to take a vat of bubbling green goo

and pour it spectacularly all over Seraphina's head. Crushes her every time.

⁓⁓ *Assignment: Create a Monster to Battle* ⁓⁓

Take one of your challenges, and let's turn it into an entity to defeat or morph into an ally. Notice its weakness. They all have weaknesses. Think about your Superpowers that can help you battle that enemy. What is the best time for you to bring it to battle? Use humor to take away a little bit of its oomph and demystify. Usually our monsters have a glimmer of ourselves or reflect some truth that we would like to avoid. The more you understand the monster, the more likely you are to rise above. You may be dealing with terrible tragedy, traumatic events, or serious illness. Only you can determine what it means to "rise above," as this can take many forms.

Posse Talk: Identifying Your Allies

Allies come in many forms. You may have friends, family, online buddies, or other people that you trust to support you. Perhaps you may not immediately be able to think of anyone that you would trust as your ally in your health quest, no problem. Developing a support system and a team may evolve throughout the quest. Part of your strength might come from a spiritual ally or your personal faith. I would like you to list three people (or entities) that you would like to have as allies. One of your allies might be analogous to my "White Angel," the little voice inside my head that talks back to the negative thoughts we all harbor.

Another way to garner support for your quest is to join an online group of people who share interests or are working on similar issues. One of the positives from social media is the ability to connect even if you don't have an immediate social circle. You can join our online support community of other avatar drivers who are also embracing a gaming approach to personal evolution, all encouraging each other on the journey to "feel good again." You'll find these links in the appendix; within these groups, you can get your questions answered and find people who will help lift you to your higher self.

—ᵛ⁄— *Assignment* —ᵛ⁄—

Reach out to someone who would be surprised to hear from you. No agenda, just touch base and say hello or even just give a smile.

Conjure Your Creative Champion

I totally love this part. You are going to design the look and feel of the little person in your head. What are they like? The main outcome here will be for you to love your hero and be able to conjure up their picture on a moment's notice!

Shape of…?

Humanoid, animal, alien, cowboy, cartoon, manga, celebrity, historical figure—the main idea is to let your imagination run wild until you find a figure with whom you resonate. Your hero might be a miniature version of you with all your future supercharged powers. Details, details, details! You really need to know exactly what your hero is wearing. What kind of "do" are they sporting? Do they have a sidekick? What are they never seen without? Minutia is important because you are going to need to be able to see that hero as clearly as you see your hand in front of your face. It's part of the program; just go with it. I recommend that you try and draw your hero; you can use the internet to help you find pictures and get ideas.

What are they driving?

Every good hero needs a jaw-dropping way to get around! Is it a car, motorcycle, hovercraft, jet? How about some kind of space vehicle? Make it awesome; it's got all the bells and whistles.

Do you hear what I hear?

What does your hero sound like? Does he or she have a battle cry? Do they have some funny sound they make right before they vanquish the enemy? Does their vehicle have a sound? Absolutely must have a theme song, no arguments. Right about now is a great time to get one of those sound effects apps on your phone so you can play some fun sound effects whenever your hero wins a battle!

Headquarters

What does it look like in your head? Remember that show *I Dream of Jeannie*? That is totally what headquarters looks like in my head; I always wanted to have a bottle like Jeannie. Color, decor, big awesome control panel, drapes? Once you have a clear picture of your hero and the space in your head, we're talking scoreboard!

Scorecard Samba

Now that you recognize yourself for the player that you are, time to embrace the idea of doing a little scorekeeping to motivate yourself. Open your mind to the momentum that can be created by a fun victory dance and reward. Just a little surge of dopamine to push you forward. This can happen in a techie or a non-techie way. As with everything, there's an app for that. At the push of a button, get a fantastic sound effect that can cheer you on. I like the app Big Button Box, there's everything from a party horn to a cracking whip to keep you motivated and give you a little power boost. I recognize this may sound silly, but until you try it, you can't really believe how well it works. Applications for Android and iPhone include Habitica and SuperBetter; both create gamified to-do lists. Earn badges and points as you check off items on your list. If you're not a techie, that is totally fine too. The non-tech equivalent is some sort of victory dance, exclamation, hand gesture—it could be pumping your fist with a yes! Personally, I enjoy a victory dance, here's the link http://

www.sunnygmd.com/sunnys-victory-dance/. I have not let my kids in on this, because they would be mortified to know that the general public could see my silly little (totally awesome) victory dance.

Not only do you need a way to celebrate, you also need a scorecard. Simple. A 3 x 5 card works just great, or a scoreboard app on your phone can be fun and has the bonus of having a timer as well. Shoot, wear a plastic wristband and decorate it with a hash mark each time you score. Another critical part of this exercise is imagining that little person in your head doing a victory dance. Work with me here, a perspective shift is an important part of the process. Trust that it will become clear, Padawan Learner, how this will take you to a whole new level as you reinvent yourself!

⤳⟋⟍⤆ *Assignment* ⤳⟋⟍⤆

Time for a victory dance! Get up off that thing and dance! Come on!

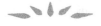

Chapter 5
Mental Preparation and Practice

Can the nuts and bolts of habit change become super sexy? Maybe, maybe not, but fortunately, hacks exist, and once you add some spice to the game, habit change can actually be fun. Here you'll find tools; look for those that resonate with your personal style. And that is important. The key elements necessary to create profound medical wellness transformation are:

- a starting point
- a vision
- a plan
- tools to get there

You have a starting point. You have a vision. You have a plan.

"You have brains in your head. You have feet in your shoes. You can steer yourself any direction you choose. You're on your own. And you know what you know. And YOU are the one who'll decide where to go…"

—Dr. Seuss

So… how to get there? Need to go to our local habit outfitter for munitions and supplies for the quest.

A Trick of the Mind

It is important that our brain buys into what we're doing here. Perception is 99% of reality. We can't always control what happens to us; we *can* control how we respond and our interpretation of events. In order to transform into Future You, you will need to spend time in your brain working with your hero embedding Future You into your avatar's wiring system. One critical concept essential to becoming "change-able" is developing your hero identity daily. As we transform slowly into our future selves, we need the neurological habit of accessing our most powerful abilities. Spending a few minutes of intention with your hero every day develops the brain connections that make conjuring the hero up when you need assistance something that comes naturally. Straight talk here. You can't skip the daily training and expect this to really work. Without the daily training, this becomes another book trying to get you to change your habits. Have those worked before for you? It may seem strange, uncomfortable, and uncharacteristic for you to intentionally take some time out of your busy day and perform this exercise. Just go with it.

Hero Training: Daydream Your Way to Future You

Daily hero training is simple; all you really need is a quiet place where you won't be disturbed. For maximum results, consider using headphones with relaxing music or a recording of binaural beats. Binaural beats can deepen meditative experiences by helping your brain waves synchronize to a more receptive frequency; by using headphones, each ear receives a slightly different tone. Immerse yourself in this training. The beats may help you move faster in the process. While you perform this exercise, slow deep breathing will activate your parasympathetic nervous system, help you de-stress and make your brain more open to suggestion.

Get into a comfortable position—consider using a progressive muscular relaxation exercise in which you sequentially contract and relax the muscles in your body beginning with your toes and moving up to your head—to get in a nice receptive state. Conjure up your hero. Use detail in your fantasy. Make your hero everything wonderful in your eyes. Clothing, tools and/or weapons—and seriously, SHOES. Where are they?

Remember headquarters? Your hero lives in an amazing place, your dream room. This fantastic room is in your head, and the large picture windows in the front give a view of everything in your line of sight. Here lies the control module that allows your hero to move your body. Part of your daily meditation requires you to visualize your hero making your body move simply using knobs or a joystick. Remember Harold and his avatar Susan? Through the game they came to understand themselves as two parts of a whole. Harold was Susan's hero, and when they began to work together, magic happened in their game. Time to connect with your hero. As your hero moves the joystick to lift your arm, actually lift your arm; do this for all of your arms and legs. The hero is in control. Your higher self, who is driven by the vision of your future, in which you are not just feeling good, but feeling great!

Key components of this daily session include clarity of process and expectation of success. You can't just "feel good" or positive about your training. The process must be crystal clear, and the expectation victory. Currently there is great interest in how we motivate ourselves, and the visualization of the process increases the likelihood that we will follow through physically. In a recent study printed in the September 2016 article in the *Journal of Health Psychology*, the authors concluded that "future clarity was positively associated with the inclination of participants to consume healthy food, abstain from cigarettes, participate in physical activity, and experience positive emotions." So the idea of daydreaming your way to your future self actually has research supporting it; practically too good to be true. Woo woo your way to wonderful. I like it.

Conjure up one of your repetitive negative thoughts and give it an adversary's body. I mentally pull up one of my adversaries, the Evil Clock. It says "no time, no time, no time, not enough time." Who can my hero bring in to help battle it? The joystick moves and a gold embossed planner flies off the shelf, immediately growing to 10 times its original size, sprouting arms and legs, and wielding an axe that smashes the Evil Clock. I love that planner. Now in my fantasy, I see myself going to my planner and entering in the things I need to do, making time for the things that are important to me. Spend anywhere from five to 30 minutes imagining battles, seeing your hero be victorious, and then seeing yourself making the choices you want to make and engaging in the habits you would like to cultivate, surrounded by the people, places, and things that are important to Future You. Feel yourself running that 5K, waking up with a bounce in your step, rocking your to-do list, winning the little struggles, sharing with others how you transformed your health and teaching them to do the same. Completing the movie by seeing Future You share with others how to transform themselves helps solidify the change within. Your fantasy sharing could take place at a large venue such as a convention, or it might be coffee with friends, just make sure it's part of your daily fantasy. This blockbuster movie will change your life if you consistently watch it daily.

Holding that vision *supported by a clear process* is essential, as it gives your subconscious a target and a path to follow. I work with clients in small groups, guiding them through a transformative process over eight weeks. To sign up, visit www.sunnygmd.com/feel-good-again-book-resources. To solidify the image of the participant's future vision, participants actually receive a digital video that incorporates pictures of their personal version of Future You, helping them easily call it up in their mind's eye. You could do a digital or physical vision board instead, simply by making a slide show of meaningful images or a poster board with a collage of pictures.

Is It Live or Is It Memorex?

Here's a revealing exercise. You and I are going to the grocery store together. We get to the fruit and vegetable aisle. You start to worry because you notice that squirrely, untamed look in my eye. Maybe it's the fact that I'm looking around to see if anybody is watching. I pick up the plumpest, yellowest lemon in all of Whole Foods and start to sing the *Chariots of Fire* theme song as I slowly bring it up toward my face. Time slows down to a crawl as you realize that your friend is about to take a honking big bite of that lemon right there, in the middle of Whole Foods in front of everybody, without buying it first. You scream "Nooooo!" as you see juice from that lemon exploding all over my wickedly grinning face…. And then…. You get too close and suddenly, into your open mouth comes a big squish of lemon! It is the tangiest taste you have ever experienced. Your mouth is watering like crazy, Heck, just writing this, my mouth is watering.

And that's the point. Now, you may never go with me to Whole Foods, but at least you understand the powerful effect fantasy has on our body physiology. My brain didn't know that wasn't real, it thought lemon was coming, and it created the appropriate response.

Within our brain, the difference between real and imagined is blurry. Memories can be manipulated creatively, and we can use this to our advantage. If you think of your average mood as created by our reactions to our thoughts, then how often we think certain thoughts and how we respond becomes more important. If we could attach each thought to a happiness or contentment gauge, we might be able to take the average of all those to determine our basic average "Happiness Measure."

So what are the variables within that equation? They are the number of times we have the thoughts and how we feel at the time. What if we were working on intentionally spending time in daydreams in which our hero made fantastic things happen in our lives, or our hero helped us to reevaluate and redefine a negative thought? What if this was actually planned into our day? Our mind doesn't truly know the difference between real and imagined, so we're having a bunch of little victories when we do this. Your daily hero training will make a difference in how you feel and your mood. It's physiology. Give it one month and judge for yourself.

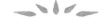

Chapter 6

Habit Boot Camp

We've got the woo woo. Now for the work. We don't often think of ourselves as animals, but that's really what we are. A puppy can be trained, and so can you. Your hero can be the benevolent trainer, kind of like a parent training up a child. The key here is frame of reference. Throughout this program, you will utilize the concept of your hero, who can be thought of as your higher self, directing the change. It's like the watcher with an attitude and an agenda— *your* agenda.

So what is your agenda? Getting to Future You. Moving from here to there. Designing the journey requires drawing on familiar ideas and incorporating new information. Transforming ourselves requires working with our habits: smashing the old bad ones and bringing on the good. Learned Behavior 101 follows.

Three Habit-Change Essentials

Before we get to describing technique, let's touch on some essentials. Three elements need to be present for long-term free and breezy habit change; of course you could just muscle through, but seriously, why? Can we please pick the easy way? Here are the three essential elements:

1. Accountability
2. A Kick-Butt Reason "Why"
3. Fun: Gamify! Gamify! Gamify!

Don't shirk on the fun. In fact, emphasize it. The more playful you can be and the less seriously you can take yourself, the lighter you become, and the greater the chance of defying gravity. We are trying to rise to the occasion; levity is key.

So now the nitty-gritty of habits. Pretty simple really. Generally speaking, habits consist of three parts, which gives us three possible points of action:

1. Trigger or Cue –this can be a person, place, thing, or even a thought.
2. The Habitual Inner Response (thoughts)or Outer Response (action)
3. Reward (the benefit you get from the response, or need that is filled by the action)

Identifying the three components of your habits will be easy at times; however, some inner responses, particularly negative thoughts, can be puzzlers for you and your hero. Imagine a baby as a perfect, simple, red rubber ball. Life takes a paintbrush and starts to paint, whirls and swirls, layers upon layers of history that influence what we do now. Somewhere in there was a time when a negative thought might have protected you, met a basic need, or preserved a relationship with someone else. It may be a script given to you by another player—a parent, a lover, a friend. Uncovering the origin of negative self-talk empowers a person to learn the lesson that needs to be learned and move on.

Negative internal scripts can, in a way, keep us safe. They maintain the status quo and prevent us from leveling up, particularly when leveling up is scary, or means a power shift in a relationship, or we must get uncomfortable and stretch our edges. We like comfort, and as you grow new habits, that's the challenge... getting over the discomfort of the stretch, and being there long enough to make it your new groove.

When you are playing the game with the intention of changing that internal script, your new script may not even seem believable to you at first. That's okay and expected. We're trying to develop new neural pathways, and it's uncomfortable. Starting with baby steps can help. The road between "I can't get anything done," and "I'm having productive days every day" requires multiple steps and making a track record so you see that you can progress. The first step would be something simple, like getting one single thing done. Score! Planning one task daily and completing it. Schwing! Tiny victories pointing you in the direction of Future You.

Think back to Harold, when he had to help his avatar overcome her sweets addiction. There were a lot of steps in the process. He had incorporated into his plan identifying cues for the behavior, figuring out what needs were met by the behavior, and then substituting something else that met the need. Similarly, this program begins with personal introspection and evaluation to identify all the pixelated habits that make up your life—then we can make a game out of optimizing avatar function. Right about now, you're probably ready to do a little bonsai cultivation of your habits, and good news, there are plenty of successful strategies. Time to pick a few that you like and use them in your game.

Starting with a little letting go… wouldn't we all like to release behaviors that aren't helping our avatars level up!?

Ditching Problematic Habits

Which aspect of your habit do you need to change to make letting go of that habit easy? The trigger? The environment? The response?

Alter the Trigger: Strategies

- **Physical environment change**. Put the cookies where we can't see them—better yet, don't even buy the cookies. Honestly, the less willpower necessary, the better.
- **Minimize the need for willpower**. Anything you can do to remove choices that take you down the wrong path, do it. Studies show that throughout the day, our willpower can weaken. Need to plan, especially when we are dealing with evening habits.
- **Change the habitual pattern of movement in your environment**. Walk through a different door where you can't see the cookies. If coming home is a trigger, make an activity plan for arrival home.

Alter the Habit: Inner Response

- **Change the trigger's meaning**. Sometimes you can't avoid or remove the triggers. This can happen when the trigger is a person. For instance, maybe there's someone whose presence leads you to pound yourself a bit with negative self-talk, or feel anxious. Perhaps you have an abusive family member. We can't change what others do or say, but we can change how we interpret and react to them.
- **Inject humor**. Give your nemesis a theme song. Maybe every time they walk up, you are hearing the Darth Vader theme in your head. Imagine them very small with a squeaky little

voice, shooting tiny little arrows at you, which bounce off your wonderfully thick skin. Picture your hero masterfully engaging and defusing them.

- **Rewrite your internal script about the trigger.** When you're feeling good (*not* triggered) write down a positive imaginary spin on why that person acts the way they act. Maybe they got a ticket driving to work this morning. Maybe they had a difficult childhood. Maybe someone yells at them at home all evening. Maybe their spouse is sick and in the hospital. Create a fantasy that makes it not about you; they are dealing with personal frustrations and you happen to be in the line of fire. Fortunately you have your armor. Your hero can handle this.

- **Visualize success daily.** Include this trigger in your daily training with a stunning display of personal mastery over it or them. Fantasy repetition. Play, replay, and replay again. Your mind doesn't know the difference between imagined feelings of victory and the actual experience of victory. We're making a track record here, rewriting your story.

Alter the Habit and Honor Your Needs

- **Identify a new activity or response that will meet the basic need:** We do things over and over for a reason. In order to change deeply ingrained habits, it's important to identify how it helps you. How do you feel when your trigger pops up? Emotions are symptoms from our body telling us that there is a deep basic need that is not being met. (Banyan 2003) Emotions associated with habits come from a desire to fulfill basic needs; the game is to find a better way to meet those needs instead of the habit you'd like to pitch. Listening to and understanding the inner wisdom of our emotions can unlock powerful change capabilities.

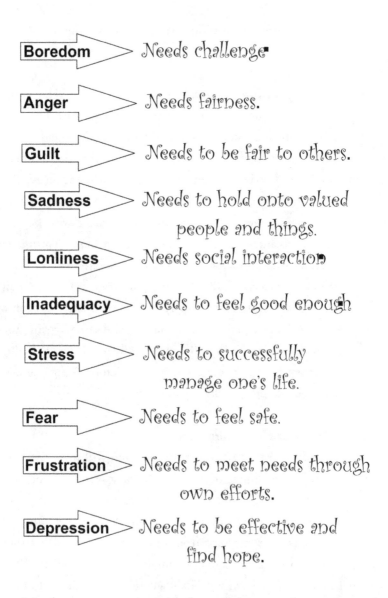

Boredom → Needs challenge

Anger → Needs fairness.

Guilt → Needs to be fair to others.

Sadness → Needs to hold onto valued people and things.

Lonliness → Needs social interaction

Inadequacy → Needs to feel good enough

Stress → Needs to successfully manage one's life.

Fear → Needs to feel safe.

Frustration → Needs to meet needs through own efforts.

Depression → Needs to be effective and find hope.

Match up your emotion with the underlying need, meet the need in a new, positive, satisfying way and the drive for the old behavior reduces.

- My end-of-the-day wine habit is definitely linked to stress: particularly time pressures and worrying how to get everything done. I switched it out for some fantastic spicy tea, which still feels like a treat, and my planner, which lets some of the air out of my freak-out balloon when I'm worried about all the things I have to do.

Adding Awesome Habits

Often easier than getting rid of bad habits, there are many ways to sneakily squish new behaviors into your life.

Techniques:

1. Habit stacking: As I have mentioned before, we're just a bunch of pixelated habits. Everything we do boils down to habit. So how can we take this fact and use it to our advantage? If you have something you do every day, it is easy to tack anew activity onto it. Take, for instance, brushing your teeth; most people do this twice a day (here's hoping). Tooth-brushing creates a golden opportunity to add something that you want to do on a regular basis to another well-established routine. Maybe you want to remember to do toe raises daily to strengthen your ankles, perhaps you need to remember to take a medication. Whatever. This technique is an effective way to create new routines, because habits love to have friends. One helpful side effect of adding new routine activities to our life is how they can crowd out those life activities that are not as healthy for us.

2. There's an app for that: if you're a smart phone user, then you can get a reminder app to help you as you initiate your new habit.

3. Habit fantasy: Include your habit in your daily hero training. Identify any obstacles and use your imagination to turn them

into a villain, an adversary, someone your hero can battle and spectacularly defeat.

4. Identify your habit change temperament. Are you "Start Small" or "Go Big?" What's your "habit change temperament?" Some folks are all or nothing. These people can really get things going, successfully biting off a big hunk of habit change. Like all of us, accountability and fun are key to helping them continue and stay on the wagon. Others feel overwhelmed by any change or really don't think it's even possible to change, and they need to start small and develop a track record.

5. Hypnotherapy: Take advantage of the power of suggestion while in a relaxed state. Hypnotherapy helps many people to shift their habits, and it's a fantastic way to connect avatar and driver, conscious and subconscious, the deeply intelligent "watcher" and the impulsive "doer." Recently published best-selling book *Reprogram Your Weight,* by Erica Flint, tells about the possibilities for tremendous results through applied hypnotherapy.

6. The Next Step: What is the tiniest next step you, as driver of your avatar, can make to take you closer to your goal? Think simple, repeatable, and easy, ludicrously easy. Toe raises or knee bends in the shower? Sure. Write it down and make a game out of how many times can you do this today or this week.

Your Deep Why

With the start of any new "program", whether it is the first day of school or the day you join the gym, comes excitement. After a while, the honeymoon ends and we grow tired of evolving, trying… we just wanna relax, already. During those plateau periods, maintaining and hanging onto the shifts you've already put into place—that is the goal. When things get tough, it's your deep reason "why" you're doing what you're doing that can give you a jumpstart.

The saying has been floated: "Get a why that can make you cry and you can move mountains." Some people have vision boards with their destiny, some people just have a picture of their child. It's not enough to just hold the vision. Deep evolution of your life requires a heart connection to the necessity of change. Do you want to live longer and be able to actually engage in life instead of watching? Take hikes and climb mountains, or even simply enjoy walking with confidence in your body? Do you want to change your children's lives? Perhaps you hold the simple goal of being there for your grandchild, going on walks holding their hand? A little story to illustrate the point:

You're standing on top of your beautiful apartment building enjoying the cityscape below when you notice, with shock, that the next building over has flames leaping out of the windows. You see that virtually all of the building is affected and people are streaming out the bottom floor. As you take it all in, you realize that there's a kid screaming on the roof. Just as quickly as you see the kid, you realize that that is *your* kid screaming. Time slows down. You look around. You see a catwalk between the buildings that is about four inches wide. You have a deep fear of heights. The flames below grow as your kid recognizes that you see her. Never on any other day would you *ever* consider walking across that catwalk. But there is only one choice; across you go to get your kid. That "why" drove you to do something extraordinary, out of character, totally unexpected, and fearless.

That kind of why can compel you to make the right choices, do the little things over and over again, and pull yourself slowly toward manifesting your higher self. Your "why" could be a strong desire or goal, like running in a race, or a trip you have been putting off because you just didn't feel well enough. Find that compelling vision and use it to help you when that little dark voice in your head asks, "Now why am I doing this?" Have your hero put in "the tape" that lays it out for you so you can clearly see your future and be inspired!

Preparation Instead of Perspiration

Something happened when Harold and Susan hit about 48. The rules of driving the avatar changed rather abruptly. Some sort of shift in neural circuitry led to alterations in recall and focus ability of the unit. Harold would send a message or instruction to Susan, for instance, object retrieval, and when they got to the proper location the recollection of the object disappeared from her mind. Also, they began the day with many ideas of things that needed to be accomplished and find very few actually completed when the sun set. This brought up anxiety levels in the avatar and Harold knew he had to find some solutions... a new challenge!

Do you ever get the end of the day and find that you have done about 10% of what you need to do? Me too. Planning is key, whether you are changing what you're eating, your activities, or even your thoughts. Planning requires discipline, and many folks find consistency in setting up a schedule and sticking to it exceptionally difficult. We tend to fall back into our routines that are familiar, basically because we're subconsciously uncomfortable changing the status quo. Our bodies and minds tend to revert to familiar, comfortable routines, because when we step out of our routines it causes anxiety. That discomfort is meant to be a protective mechanism on the most basic level. It's meant to keep us safe; however, when we're talking about the evolution of a person, playing it safe can keep us locked in a cage.

So how to get out of that cage and fly free, little birdie? It's called a planner. Call me crazy, I don't mind; this can change your life. If you don't have things planned and things written down, then you spend a lot of subconscious background energy worrying about the people, places, events, and activities to which you have committed.

Let's go ahead and make plan. Does this seem like a medical thing to you? Maybe not, but let me tell you, I spent a lot of time working with people who are stressed out, depressed, and anxious, and there is a deep commonality. An underground river of unmet personal commitments to self and others—promises we have made to ourselves, our family, our parents, our work—provides constant fuel to the subconscious mind, creating anxiety whose origin we can't quite put our finger on. This makes it a medical issue.

The physical state of stress and worry translates to a shift in the chemical balance in the body—in particular, an uptick in cortisol, which is our stress hormone. Chemical imbalances affect our emotions, our perception of pain, our bodily symptoms, our ability to sleep—the list goes on. The personal work of identifying those commitments is a topic for another book. For now, know that acknowledging the historical tiny needles in your soul and making peace, amends, retribution is hugely important for your psychological health.

Right now, let's just try and get your current commitments on the books. So maybe I'm the first doctor to tell you to get a planner and a "to do" list to offload all those things spinning in your brain, that's okay by me. Your hero needs a Zen garden in which to train, not a thicket of barbed wire. Planning your day will give you control, clarity and a sense of "I can do this thing, man!"

⇜ *Assignment* ⇜

- Set aside 10 minutes each evening to plan tomorrow.
- Write it down or put it in your phone, put it in the planner—whatever you have to do make it easy to access.
- Rinse and repeat.

The Magic of Little Things

One of my favorite books is *The Slight Edge,* by Jeff Olson. A fantastic and highly recommended read, it goes on to explain how seemingly insignificant small habits repeated on a daily basis change the trajectory of your life. For instance, how about the choice of "should I have a glass of water or a glass of a soft drink?" One decision takes you to a very different physical state when compounded over an extended period of time. In the moment, it seems like a fairly insignificant choice, and we tend to let our history and our emotions decide in the moment. If we make a habit of engaging our hero during moments like these, having planned for the decisions (because you probably can guess what's going to come at you during the day), we can start to pick the course that will propel us in the direction we want to go. These small things are "easy to do and easy to not do." Making a habit of choosing the small things that are in alignment with our future self takes us closer to that vision. Score! Booyah!

—‹›‹— *Assignment* —‹›‹—

1. Build brain buy-in through daily hero training.
2. Identify one or two habit-change strategies that feel right and will work on your most pressing issues.
3. Plan every day either on paper or electronically.
4. One thing at a time; tiny steps will take you to your goal.

TOOL KIT FOR QUEST CREATION

The shift has happened. There is no going back. Now you understand your role as the driver. Your avatar needs you to guide it to optimal function. The remainder of this manual instructs newly emerged drivers in ways to more effectively manage their avatar, beginning with executive circuitry. Every change begins in the mind, and so that is where this begins. Twist the lens and shift your perspective. You have landed in the game, and you are powerful.

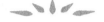

Chapter 7

The Transformation Process and Your Powerful Mind

Shift to a Challenge Mindset

On waking today, what do you think was the first thing that popped into my head? Like many of you, my wickedly long to-do list floated in front of my eyes and started spinning like a tornado in the center of my brain. Fun cartoon tornado? No, menacing, seething, dark cloud of commitments spinning out of control. Gosh, I hate it when that happens! How we manage our first thought matters. When you wake up, your body may start immediately talking to you. It may be back pain, it may be a joint aching, it may be a headache, it may be your to-do list. Whatever your stormy cloud or malevolent monster, let's figure out a way to put you in the driver's seat and shift the tide in the power struggle. Waking up and feeling immediately defeated pretty much just sucks. So let's change that.

Calling all heroes! It's time to put on your Superpower holster and engage the enemy in battle. We start by changing how we think about our big issues. Most people do not choose to have debilitating disease, pain, stressful work situations or family life, or disruption and upheaval, but they still have to decide how to manage it and choose whether they are pulled along behind the horse or riding it.

There are five steps to take when you're trying to turn your threat into a challenge and enter into the adventure:

1. **Give your nemesis a game name and** invite it into the battle arena in your mind. Be creative, use some humor. See it. Make it kinda ugly.

2. **Choose your challenge.** You are the one in control of this round; you have home-court advantage. The greatest growth comes from the most difficult personal battles. By making a decision to invite the monster into the ring, you begin the shift from a threat mindset to a challenge mindset.

3. **Arm your hero.** What are the qualities that your hero needs in order to overcome this particular challenge, and what steps will it take? Are there new skills you need? What are your best strengths that can help you meet the challenge?

4. **Visualize your battle before it happens!** Remember, at the beginning of the day, each and every day, you're watching an internal movie starring your hero, connecting with your powerful internal source of intelligence. Two minutes, five minutes, 60 minutes, however long it takes. Remember the essential parts to the movie:

a. Relaxation and connection of avatar and driver

b. Review your day and anticipate the battles. What strategies will you and your hero use? Create some battle scenes: fun, frantic, and furious. You win!

c. "A day in my life." An amazing movie of Future You long after the battle, feeling the way you want to feel, thinking what you want to think, meeting all your challenges, in the place you want to be, with the people you want to be surrounded by. You in all your glory, at the top of your game. Healthy, vibrant, seeing good things happen, helping other people to do the same thing that you have done. This should be so crystal-clear that you feel waves of happiness while you watch this movie.

5. **Get your scorecard ready and start battling!** The low-tech version is a handy-dandy 3 x 5 card, but don't forget about the high-tech versions like Habitica or "Superbetter" –get one! Make a list of things you can do to trounce the enemy.

6. **Give yourself a point for all things good.** Even the tiny things count; you get credit for something as simple as pulling yourself out of the comfort of your bed. Big wins come from adding up all the tiny little victories.

7. **At the end of the day, celebrate your scorecard.** A gratitude journal can also be very helpful. Studies have shown that keeping a daily gratitude journal can improve mood, diminish depression, and boost optimism. (Sirois FM 2016) This was the first longitudinal investigation of gratitude and what's great about gratitude. It is side-effect free. That's my kind of drug!

A helpful principle in reframing our interpretation of events and thoughts is the fact that our bodies have two principal settings. We continually balance between the "rest and digest" mode and the "fight or flight" mode. Our body feels a certain way, and we interpret those physical sensations as a "state." It is possible to use this to our advantage and reinterpret physical sensations. For instance, when we are anxious or worried we feel on edge—elevated heart rate, more sensitive, alert, jittery, our breath comes faster. Note that excitement causes the same body response. The next time you feel anxiety, try saying "I'm excited." This might sound false at first, but what you tell yourself matters.

Often an emotion accompanies physical states, and then we can use Calvin Banyan's principles mentioned earlier to try and identify what's the basic need that underlies the emotional state, and how we can meet that need.

- Boredom wants challenge
- Anger and guilt both want fairness (for self and others, to self and others)
- Sadness wants to hold onto valued things and people
- Loneliness desires relationship
- Inadequacy wants to feel good enough
- Stress wants to regain control
- Frustration wants to be able to meet personal needs through personal deeds
- Depression wants to be effective and hopeful

Self-Talk Magic

There are a lot of thoughts running around in our heads, right? Hopefully when you did your intensive mirror exercise, you identified thoughts and phrases that commonly pop up in your own head. Sadly, often our self-talk is self-defeating talk. Our habitual thoughts are just that, habits, and we can break them; most of us would like to let go of our personal browbeating, and it can be as simple as finding a new path.

Let's imagine you're at a lake house, and every day you and your family take the same grassy path down to the lake. It's the easiest way to go, so why would you take a different path? Each time you make your way to the water, the path becomes clearer, more tramped down, easier to find. This is also how our neural circuitry works. Neurons that fire together, wire together, and the more often we repeat an action or a thought, the more hardwired it becomes. Nice thing that we have "brain plasticity!" We used to think our brains didn't change a whole lot after a certain age. Now we know that you *can* change the connections in your brain. You can change habits. You can change habitual thoughts. What we need is a new path to the lake. Research on gaming theory also tells us that we activate different areas of our brain when we turn it into a game; the mundane becomes interesting and engaging. So how do we use this to our advantage?

Time to write a new script. Another opportunity to use those handy-dandy 3 x 5 cards, or the awesome app you've downloaded to make this way fun. Pick one of your personal scripts you would like to change. Maybe every time you see a grumpy checkout person at the grocery store, you play a negative script about yourself. Could be that when your in-laws criticize you or your parent brings up something from childhood (why can't they just let that go?!), you feel enraged. What about that repetitive memory that invades your mind unexpectedly? Our "auto-scripts" can lead us to dark, unfriendly places, spiraling down complete with body memories and physical sensations that have been played over and over.

This is a health issue. I have to interject that here, because I can imagine someone reading this and thinking, "What does this have to do with my health?" Emotional states create physiological changes. If we live in a constant state of sadness, sour mood, anxiety, or fight or flight, our hormone levels like cortisol and thyroid hormone and the balance of the neural messengers in the brain shift; this negatively affects our body in many ways. Additionally, our mental state of mind deeply informs whether or not we think we can do something. When we are talking about big habit change, we need to know in our core that change is possible. So if you have a little something that you have been whispering in your ear for many years, or maybe you're hearing someone else's voice whispering it in your ear, let's turn it into a monster to be squished. Just like before, you're going to:

- **give the villain a game name**
- **invite the villain to battle: your court, your rules**
- **arm your hero: the qualities your hero will use to vanquish the enemy**
- **visualize the battle in advance—grab your scorecard and enter the ring!**

Every mistake is just a mistake unless you learn from it; then it becomes a valuable life lesson. If we beat ourselves up for mistakes, we stop trying new things, and then we stop growing. So let's make more mistakes, keep growing, and figure out how to feel okay about it. At times when people are depressed, a tiny little demon in their head takes an opaque black crayon and colors on top of their thoughts, making the negative stand out, underlining blame, creating self-directed blaming thought bubbles, and rewriting current events as a tragedy, starring—ta da, right? How to get rid of the graffiti?

- Identify the thought.
- Let your hero evaluate the truth of it—is it really all the way true?
- Would you say this to a friend asking for interpretation or advice?
- In what ways has the little demon distorted the facts?

- Are you jumping to conclusions or mind-reading without hard evidence?
- Have you discounted the positive?
- Let your hero rewrite the thought in a 100% truthful way.

Let's say I wanted to stop beating myself up when I am late to an event. (Maybe being late is something I want to work on too, but let's start off with making peace with our current state.)

When I'm running late, I have the habitual thought, "I am a total flake because I can't get places on time." That's a script I would like to change. I need to analyze that statement in a fair way and find a different thought that can take its place that is really true, that I can believe, *and* that leaves me feeling okay about what is happening. In this one, I'm passing judgment on my entire being based on being a few minutes late. Not very fair. So maybe I am a "work in progress" instead of a "total flake." The "work in progress" concept is one of my favorites, because it can be applied to anything. It implies learning from doing. We will repeat history over and over again until we analyze it and adjust. Perhaps I could say to myself:

- "Running late today is going to help me figure out how to plan better." And then make a plan.
- "I completed important tasks in exchange for being on time."
- "I am so glad I was 15 minutes late, because now I know exactly how much extra time I need to get ready." Big note to self: always add 15!

Everybody's got their own insecurities. Negative thoughts plague most of us at various times in our lives. The first step to changing that script is recognizing that this is happening. I like using those 3 x 5 cards because they have two sides. Capture your negative thoughts on one side of the 3 x 5 card, and then write a rational response on the opposite side. You need to be wearing clothing with pockets to carry these around with you! Catching yourself having a negative thought is key; that split-second of recognition holds the opportunity for growth. Pull out your 3 x 5 card and read your alternative rational thought and give yourself a point on the card. See how many times you can catch yourself having that thought and reading your alternative rational thought during the day. Play your sound effect from your app or do your victory dance! Whatever makes it fun for you!

Claim Your Power

What do you do when you feel like you can't do it? It's just too much. You've never done it before, and why should you be able to do it now? You may know all the right things to do, you may even be able to write a book about all the right things to do to make yourself feel good, be happy—and still be unable to put these things into action. Fortunately for you, when you were a baby you didn't let thoughts like these get you down, so let's figure out how to manage them now. Time to claim your power.

Remember that in our initial mirror exercise, you wrote down your positive qualities, and if you had a hard time thinking of positive qualities, you used the Values in Action character survey to identify your top five power points. These are qualities you hold that have the potential to shine through in your thoughts and actions, creating positive ripples in your life and the lives of others. Owning these and expanding these will help you roll forward. These need to go on a card or poster in a place that you see every day. I would like you to be able to shut your eyes and see them, preferably to see them in action in your life. It may be difficult to clearly see these powers manifesting in your life. Use fantasy and create scenarios; you are practicing using your powers. Morning hero training gives you a boost, makes you feel better before the day even starts. Use your powers for good—your own good.

Personal growth and introspection: those two are holding hands. Since you are thinking about your Superpower Pack in the morning, identifying times when your awesome qualities come into play becomes easier. Many of us tend to downplay our positives and remember our negatives, so let's turn that upside down. Time to make it a game and see how many times your wonderfulness comes into play during the day.

The power up!
Super easy, super effective. Steps to claiming your power include:

- practice your power in the morning
- identify snapshots of time when you can use your power or you could have used your power
- use your power and score a point
- get closure: mentally recreate an event that didn't go as you would have liked, add a better ending using your power and replay at least two times: score two points!

Create a track record
It takes many people with the same idea to create a movement, and many tiny successes to create a habit. Developing a success mindset requires laying down a track record. When we are creating our track record, we start with the easiest thing possible. Something we know that we can do regularly. When your journey of discovery conjured up Future You and how you will be feeling, who will be surrounding you in what amazing place, how wonderful your health will be… all of that begins with one tiny little cornerstone habit.

It's critical that you choose something you can successfully do and track. That's why we call it a track record; you will be showing yourself your ability to make a tiny commitment and keep it. We are starting to increase the good, bringing you the bounty with a tiny drop of positivity. Your cornerstone habit might be as simple as reading a daily affirmation, smiling at a stranger, waiting five minutes before you get seconds—choose anything that moves you a tinge closer to that Future You.

⟶ᴗᵎᵎᵎᵎ⟵ *Assignment* ⟶ᴗᵎᵎᵎᵎ⟵

Pick the smallest of habits. The simpler, the better. Something that brings a touch of joy. I am not talking a daily run. More like wrestling with your dog and sending it a whole bunch of love. (Pet interactions will give you extra points, because they actually give you love back!) Make it easy. Use the habit stacking technique. You have to wake up every day, so maybe when you wake up every day, read your 3 x 5 card with your Superpower Pack on it. Have it right there by your bedside. I like for people to continue with the cornerstone habit exercise for several days, preferably a week, keeping written or recorded score somewhere that they can look back on.

What's Your Power Source and How Do You Plug into It?

Are you one of those folks who can immediately identify the best way to personally recharge? Do you intentionally create moments that allow you to regroup, breathe, let go of work, drop the electronics, and release your psychic connection to all your commitments? Personally, I find that when electronic tragedy strikes and my phone and computer are rendered disabled by a power outage (and I have gone through the stages of denial, anger, bargaining, and depression), when I get to acceptance, I feel an overwhelming wave of relief. Quite a phenomenon. While imposed by the universe, that sense of letting go that comes with the inconvenience shows me that I probably need to try and figure out a way to make that happen on my own.

When you want to recharge and calm the chaos within your mind, identifying activities, places, and states that have brought you the most peace and rejuvenation in the past can help. A life review of sorts, the goal here is to gather *all* the potential tools by carefully considering each part of your life and remembering where you have found solace. Interestingly, when we conduct our life review in this way, we also can identify times in our game of life when our avatar bought into booby-traps or was led astray to use coping skills that really led to demotion or a lower level in our proverbial quest.

Where and when did you experience the most profound happiness? Who was around you? What kind of things were you doing? What has brought you the most pleasure during your life—true pleasure, without the kind of emotional extra baggage that requires amputation by a therapist? Sometimes we forget things that brought us joy when we were young, or we think we can't really do those things anymore. One of the most profound opportunities for joy is to regain the experience of doing something you loved and let go of long ago, maybe because there just wasn't enough time, money, whatever. How can we sneak back in the things that elevate us to our best selves?

When speaking of how to achieve profound relaxation and rest, any discussion would be incomplete to leave out yoga, tai chi, meditation, artistic endeavors, music, you name it. An artistic flow state can give a person a big battery boost, even though it may not seem "restful." By achieving a true flow state where one balances on the edge of one's abilities, the individual is drawn into that artistic space where time stands still and the outside world goes away. These kinds of activities will help you balance the sympathetic and parasympathetic nervous system. So if you're one of those all-work-and-no-play folks, that might be something you want to reconsider! We knew we needed to play when we were kids. Why did we forget this?

—✦— *Assignment* —✦—

Identify three activities that put you in a "flow state." Put one of these in your planner. Connect with someone who also enjoys doing this activity.

Affirmations and Awe

Boosting the good requires intention. Affirmations are phrases that embody and describe our Future Self in the form of our true self, our soul's magnetic North. Don't be tempted to skip the easy things. Sometimes they turn out to be the most important things. This is reinforcing your Superpower Pack as you do in your morning hero training, but I think being effusive and all-inclusive in a few well-written sentences (that may keep changing) imbues your hero with a vision of their destiny, as written by you. So easy, yet so easy; yep… no excuses. Read these every day, and give yourself a point!

Awe-some therapy? How about the research study that showed the positive health effects of experiencing awe? Measuring one of the powerful inflammatory substances in our body, interleukin six, researchers at UC Berkley showed that people who had more daily experiences of awe (such as soaking up a breathtaking view, becoming immersed in music or creative endeavors, tree-gazing, taking a hike) had lower blood levels of this inflammatory substance. (Stellar JE 2015). This makes me want to run outside, lie down in the grass, and look up at the big tree in my yard. Or, depending on the time of year, snow. Anybody for a snow angel?

—✦— *Assignment* —✦—

Engage in Awe Therapy today. Look for it. Seek it out. This could be as simple as googling amazing nature photographs, or holding your kid's hand and thinking about how tiny it is or used to be.

Drive Yourself to Distraction

Sometimes, we need to deal with our stuff; sometimes we need to avoid our stuff. When we are talking about diminishing the negative influences in our life, avoidance can be good. This applies to triggers that take you to habits you want to get rid of, relationships that suck away your happiness, places you know are no good for you. Strategizing how to do this requires that you think about it beforehand. You made an initial inventory of your habits and things you would like to change; some can be managed through simple avoidance and planning ahead. If you're trying to drink less alcohol, don't hang out with folks who drink too much. Or rather, choose to hang out with people that have the outlook and habits you envision for yourself. Studies show that our habits and health tend to reflect that of the people with whom we spend the most time. (Christakis NA 2007) (Watt RG 2014) (Sawka KJ 2015)

Chapter 8

The Transformation Process and Gut Health

Elimination Diet for Identifying Mystery Substances that Make You Ill

Leveling up and feeling good again requires support of the avatar by getting rid of exposures that negatively affect function. Could be food, toxins, people, places, the house you live in, stuff you put on your face—a lot of possibilities here. Fortunately, we have built-in systems to detoxify and protect ourselves from infectious invaders, to repair our DNA when our inner mechanic goes a little astray, and to keep our body in tip-top condition. However, these mechanisms can't run well without the right, supportive building blocks—i.e., your basic nutrition—and avoidance of the substances that cause damage. Harold figured it out... avatar care comes first. So how do we figure out what's hurting us vs.

what turns us into the Energizer Bunny? Sometimes it's simple. Every time I have a milkshake, I'm racing to the bathroom. Other times it takes a bit more work. Since you're reading this book, you might fall into the latter category.

When it comes to fuel, you want to find what works best for you personally. Food causes different kinds of reactions. You've heard of allergy to gluten, which is called celiac disease, and this is a classic allergy. The body makes immunoglobulins against proteins found in gluten. Some people are not allergic to gluten, but their body is *sensitive* to gluten. This is not a classic allergy like celiac disease, but that doesn't mean it doesn't exist. When we are wondering what fuel is best for our body, the simplest way to identify what works is to go on an elimination diet. This is where you limit your intake initially to foods that rarely cause reactions in people, and then slowly, one at a time, add the removed foods back to see how your body responds. There are quite a few popular books describing how to do an elimination diet. It can be used for autoimmunity, allergies, fibromyalgia… everybody calls it different things, but let's be real here, it is just an elimination diet.

The foods initially removed are those that most commonly cause reactions, and they are: gluten, dairy, soy, and soy products, shellfish, refined sugar (white sugar, high fructose corn syrup, brown sugar, sucrose, etc.), alcohol, red meat, chocolate, coffee, soft drinks, tea, corn, eggs, and sometimes nuts and legumes. Let me emphasize that this is not a forever diet! This is a means to an end of figuring out why you feel funky bad. Your avatar will thank you. After that initial washout period, foods are gradually added back in, tracking the body's response. A properly done elimination diet with adequate nutritional support can affect:

- intensity of pain in the body and joints
- mood

- stomach complaints
- foggy brain and focus
- fibromyalgia
- neurological complaints
- ADD/ADHD
- autoimmune conditions
- inflammatory disorders
- and even more...

Powerful. But the key is doing it right. Many people come to me having tried an elimination diet and saying it did not work. Often folks add food back in too quickly to really identify sensitivities. Not easy, but you only want to do this once, so do it right. When you add foods back in, only add one food at a time, giving yourself five to six days with constant monitoring of symptoms in a diary to see if it really causes sensitivity. The reason we give it six days is because sometimes it takes up to five days to see subtle sensitivities. If you've already added in another food, you will not know what caused the problem. On my website you can download a version of an elimination diet for free, or you can look for this wonderful book, *The Elimination Diet: Discover the Foods That Are Making You Sick and Tired - and Feel Better Fast,* by Tom Malterre MS, CN and Alissa Segersten, which includes a lot of amazing recipes and a meal plan.

Increasing the Good: Vegetables, Slowing down and Food Reintroduction

If you have started an elimination diet, you're probably eating a lot of vegetables. Vegetables are magic; the rainbow of colors gives nutrients that are required for our bodies to function well. Some people tell me that they *thought* they were eating a lot of vegetables before they started the elimination diet, and then they realized what "a lot of vegetables" really means. Volume veggies. Eat a salad bowl the size of your head every day if possible… no, don't eat the bowl, eat the huge salad it holds. (This makes me think of Cookie Monster—he would eat the salad bowl. Let's imagine us eating the salad just like "Cookie" would, with all the sound effects.)

Increasing the good in terms of meals means slowing down, enjoying your food, sitting down with people you enjoy, and creating a new personal food culture. Most of us are in such a hurry; we eat in the car, on the go, while we are taking a run. It's crazy. For good digestion, a person needs to smell the food, anticipate the food. Digestion begins with salivation and looking forward to the meal. You'll be able to digest better if you use this knowledge and take time to make meals almost ritualistic. Chewing to liquefaction can actually make you feel better. Meals are not the time to have discussions of wicked politics; that just messes everybody up. Heated discussions during meals allow your sympathetic nervous system to take over; that, my friend, is fight or flight, not rest and digest.

Speaking of digesting, if you embarked upon an elimination diet, there comes a time when you must start to add back in the foods that you removed. As mentioned before, it's critical to the process that you *slowly* bring those foods back onto the menu. The only way to recognize sensitivities is to give each food those five to seven days to see if you react. Food sensitivities do not necessarily show up as a stomachache. They can show up as a headache, joint aches, muscle pain, foggy brain, low energy, any and all of those nonspecific symptoms could be related to what you eat. So if during the reintroduction phase you develop symptoms, remove the food again for a week and then try again and see what happens. That's the best way to gauge non-allergic food sensitivity.

Adding the good in terms of digestion can also mean considering taking an enzyme supplement and a probiotic to help support the happy family living in your gut. Most folks who are trying to use an elimination diet to reduce symptoms would benefit from four to six weeks of a gut-healing supplement in addition to the enzymes and probiotics. Talk with your naturopath or functional medicine provider to get suggestions on gut-healing supplements. The goal is to heal the gut, so that only desired substances get through the gut wall.

When our gut wall is leaky and allows unwanteds to sneak in between the cells, those substances meet up with our immune system. You may remember that most of our immune system (lymphatic tissue) is lining the walls of our gut, waiting to determine if substances getting through the gates are friend or foe. When these immune cells meet up with substances that would not ordinarily get across the gut barrier, they decide whether or not they need to call out the troops to clear them out of the body. The problem is when a danger signal is activated in response to a molecule that looks like something normally in our body. That creates a situation where our body activates the immune system against the self: autoimmunity, autoinflammation. Healing the gut by using enzymes, probiotics, healthy whole foods without pesticides, and gut-healing supplements helps heal the leaky gut and make you feel better. Staying the course with an elimination diet? Hard thing for people to do. Take a gaming approach; it becomes more fun and easier.

⁓ Assignment ⁓

Eat the rainbow today. Remember from your science classes? ROYGBIV. Get every color. Or maybe you could go for volume veggies today! How many cups of vegetables can you squeeze in? Here's a hint: steamed greens. Can you get in six to nine cups?

Your Little Friends, the Microbiota

Remember, you are simply the largest organism in your personal cloud. Taking care of the cloud should be a very high priority if you're trying to feel your best. Part of your posse is your microbiota. These little friends need tender loving care. Everything that falls down your gullet affects them, and they affect how you feel. Several ways to care for your little buddies: avoid pesticides, consume probiotic food such as fermented vegetables, limit sugar, limit antibiotics whenever possible, and make sure you have enough fiber in your diet.

Fantastic Fiber

So what is the magic in vegetables? A good bit of it is the fiber. Your avatar will last longer and better if you give it fiber daily. If you go to PubMed and search online, you will find a lot of published studies trying to tease out its benefits. A study published in the November, 2016 issue of the journal *Nutrients* looked at fiber intake and cardiovascular risk. Participants with higher dietary intake from legumes as well as fruits and vegetables had lower risk of cardiovascular disease. Intake of fiber coming from nuts or grains did not have the same effect. (Mirmiran P 2016) Fiber affects glucose levels, elimination, how much extra weight we carry around, and much more. I think everyone should consider adding some extra to their diet; it helps to feed your microbiome, and helps with elimination. A little caution here, however, because adding fiber can cause bloating and discomfort. A little at a time is the best way to go. Work with your medical provider to identify what is the best way to increase your fiber beyond a wonderful diet with lots of vegetables and fruits. As a general rule, soluble fiber (dissolves in liquid) slows the food going through you and insoluble fiber—roughage—speeds it up.

⁓⭒⭒⭒⁓ *Assignment* ⁓⭒⭒⭒⁓

Learn how to use the wonderful resource PubMed.gov. Are you wondering about the latest published research regarding the health advice that Aunt May just gave you? PubMed is a free resource available to everyone where you can find articles to help guide your health quest. If the articles don't make sense to you, consider taking them to your doctor or your healthcare provider so they can check them out and interpret. You might be able to bring great information that they have not yet seen that could be beneficial in their practice. Here is a link (also in appendix): <u>https://www.ncbi.nlm.nih.gov/pubmed</u>. Type in "fiber and cardiovascular disease" in the search box and see if you can find the article I referenced. Power to the people!

Chapter 9

The Transformation Process and Balance

Parasympathetic-Sympathetic Seesaw

Nice being at the top of the food chain; most of us don't have to worry about being eaten by a tiger the way our distant ancestors did. While our living situations have evolved, our physiology remains quite primitive. Our bodies constantly work to balance the two parts of our autonomic nervous system: the parasympathetic and the sympathetic. In short, the sympathetic speeds us up, puts us on edge, and gets us ready, and the parasympathetic slows us down. We must have both, but they need to be in balance. Your sympathetic nervous system keeps you safe during times of danger and puts you on your toes when it is time to run, but it also tends to end up on overdrive in our overstimulated, overcommitted, ridiculously busy world. When the sympathetic nervous system is in charge, we stay in a low-level version of "fight or flight," and all the "rest and digest" components of the parasympathetic nervous system are down-regulated. Bummer. Any processes unnecessary for the serpentine run through adversarial fire to safety are dampened. This decreases and messes with our libido, ability to easily digest foods, reproductive hormone balance, cellular repair machinery, and normal sleep-wake cycling, to name a few. When fight or flight is in charge, we release more cortisol, our natural stress hormone, which does many things including releasing glucose from cells for instant energy. This is great when you need to sprint, but over time high glucose levels contribute to the development of insulin resistance, diabetes, and feeling bad. Yikes!

Creating this balance in your life may seem out of reach. That's okay. We are where we are, and the idea is just to take little steps forward. A whole lot of variables contribute to your autonomic balance, and you already familiar with some of these: getting good sleep, eating well, being with community, exercising—not rocket science. As a society, we find it difficult to find the time and make ourselves do what we need to do. The low-level anxiety that comes with that persistent mini fight-or-flight experience happening in our control system leaves us constantly wide-eyed and panicking underneath cool exteriors. In order to regain command, we have to boost that parasympathetic nervous system. Fortunately, there are specific exercises that will improve the nervous system balance, helping you feel more in control and able to do the things you know that you should do.

One measure of nervous system balance is heart rate variability (HRV). Heart rate variability is little tiny shifts in the measurement between heartbeats caused by the push and pull of the two parts of the autonomic nervous system. Many in the medical arena are looking at correlation between heart rate variability and common medical problems. Studies in the growing field have recognized an association between worse outcomes in diabetes and increased risk of sudden cardiac death, (Hottenrott K 2006), as well as an association with high heart rate variability and improved cardiovascular performance and fitness. (JG 2106) Avoidance of sudden cardiac death might just be your really good reason "why." (Back to the basic idea that if you don't have a really good reason why, you're not going to keep doing a random new behavior.) Avatar drivers need to keep revisiting their motivation to keep their avatar running well, understanding that what drives us shifts as we evolve. Avoiding a heart attack might be enough motivation for you, but it's so much more fun to incorporate the concept of driving your avatar to rock the game of life and vanquish your challengers. Now of course you all realize that the point of having a blast while climbing up the Game Level Pyramid (a game that is a whole lot better when you get to play with an able body) is to keep it "able" as long as possible.

How can we impact our heart rate variability to keep our bodies able? Exercise, tai chi, meditation, hypnosis, slow deep breathing exercises, and guess what? There's an app for all of those. (That joke is getting old, sorry!) Heart rate variability can be accurately measured by the camera on your phone just by pressing your finger to the camera and using the appropriate application. If you are a non-techie, not to fret, slow deep breathing and relaxation therapy don't require technology. They require practice. Practice requires motivation, motivation comes from:

- initiation of the practice (sometimes you just have to start)
- enjoyment of the practice
- seeing results (measurement, scorecard)
- your deep "why"

How can we make slow deep breathing and relaxing fun? Many respond by saying, "Yes I would love to do that, but I just don't have time."

Clearly, we need a fun game that works!

—᭡᭡᭡— *Assignment* —᭡᭡᭡—

Time to invent your own challenges. Some ideas:

- How many times during the day can I remember to take slow deep breaths (one point for each)?
- Use a timer or an intermittent bell on your phone (I love the app Mindfulness Bell) to bring yourself back to your breath (one point for each time you're already in the slow breathing zone).
- Set up an arrangement with an ally who can shoot you a surprise text during the day; if you've done some deep breathing in the past hour before they text you, that's a point.

This is meant to be easy. Life does not need to change for you to do this, but your life will change if you take this and run with it. Easy to do, easy to not do. Your choice. Your why.

Happy Place Cultivation

We live in a fast society. Walking fast, talking fast, overscheduled. (Maybe it's just me… not!) What does this mean for our bodies? As animals, we have a pretty neat rudimentary system in place to keep us safe. When we feel threatened, our nervous system goes into "get me out of here" mode—in contrast to that trip to Hawaii, when the body's intelligence puts us in "rest and digest" mode.

What happens to us when we combine spinning brain—trying to keep all the balls in the air—and an overscheduled day with persistent worrisome thoughts or anxieties? It's a tiger around every corner, baby. Spending a lot of time in fight or flight gets tiring, and can make us sick. Persistent activation of our sympathetic nervous system can depress our resilience, immunity, ability to process food, increase our anxiety, and can create a downward spiral. When you can't change your schedule, what can you do?

We all need an immediately accessible happy place. There is a way to cultivate it. The basic idea is that you get yourself into a very relaxed state by using slow deep breathing and envisioning an uber-wonderful environment of your choice; associate it with a scent and a song, (both of which are portable), practice it, and voilá: mobile happy place.

Ingredients:

- Your favorite music. I would suggest some kind of mellow groove for happy place cultivation.
- A smell or essential oil you like—this is all about you :-)
- A spot you can totally relax. This might be the bath, maybe a comfy chair.
- Consider adding a super-soft blanket, hot water bottle, or something of the like.

The upfront effort is worth it. Go to your perfect happy place 10 minutes daily for one week. Use slow deep breathing, visualize all the best places and events, or clear your mind and focus on the breath. Whatever is most relaxing—it is your happy place, after all! Then you can back off the frequency, but the more you practice, the more effective this will be. Next you can take your show on the road. Armed with a song on your phone and the essential oil tucked somewhere like your pocket, you're set. Try going to your happy place at work. It should get easier and easier to activate the rest and digest, soothe and slowdown part of you.

—⚜— *Assignment* —⚜—

Make yourself a mobile happy place.

The Magic of a Good Sleep and How to Get It

People do not function well without good sleep; there's a chicken and egg question when it comes to sympathetic dominance and sleeping. Improving the parasympathetic output should, in theory, improve sleeping, and sleeping better, should, in theory, improve your heart rate variability or autonomic balance. Our body functions best when we have a relatively constant wake-up time, even on the weekends. Shift work? You may need a job-ectomy. In health terms it is better to consistently be a day or night person. Sometimes there's just no choice, but either way, "sleep hygiene" concepts can help you maximize your sleep. Components of setting yourself up for sleeping are:

- a consistent bedtime and a consistent wake time
- a dark bedroom without any blinky, flashy charger lights
- no pets in the bedroom
- either a quiet room or white noise to cover up any possibly wakeful sounds
- no TV, no electronics, nothing in the bedroom that will wake you up when you look at it
- if you have to have your cell phone in your bedroom, put it on a nighttime setting that has a low light
- use the bed only for sleeping and intimacy, not for reading or watching television
- daily exercise, but not in the two hours before bed
- stay well-hydrated during the day, but discontinue fluids for two hours before bed, because concentrated urine can be a bladder irritant and wake you up
- train your internal clock
- consider wearing amber glasses for an hour before going to sleep
- full-spectrum "happy light" for thirty minutes upon waking
- if you run cold, consider sleeping with a hot water bottle

- low-dose melatonin can be helpful for some to reset their internal clock

There is a well-established way to improve sleep and reset your clock. If you have health or psychiatric issues, you may want to discuss this with your doctor, because it definitely involves a little bit of fatigue. The basic idea is that you:

- estimate how long you are actually asleep—call that X hours
- set a wake-up time *in stone*
- at first, make your bed time X hours before your wake up time.

You won't get all the sleep you need; this works because you become a little sleep-deprived. Begin by setting your consistent wake-up time, and then figure out how long you are *actually sleeping* at night. For instance, if you usually lay in bed for four hours and sleep for four hours, you set your wake-up time at seven, you will go to bed at three in the morning so you get four hours of sleep. Doing this, you will accumulate sleep debt; napping is not allowed in order for this to work. When you are sleeping 80% of the time that you are lying in bed, the next night you can move your bedtime 30 minutes earlier. Over the course of several days to several weeks, people can reset their clocks this way.

Keep track of your sleep. Use a FitBit or some other personal tracking application. Little tiny gains otherwise go unnoticed. Usually when sleep starts to change, it is gradual. In order to give yourself credit, you have to track it. Scorecard, baby.

Work and Play

A quick nod here to the idea of balancing work and play. I see what happens when people reduce their commitments. Unfortunately, it creates a vacuum, a black hole that tries to suck you into more activity.

You got rid of one commitment, and then the next day someone is asking you to be on the board. As difficult as it can be, the word "no" is a must for the repertoire of the balanced person. Practice it in the mirror. Learn to say it in a kind manner. No highly productive person can create a balanced life without understanding and wielding the power of "no" effectively.

Chapter 10

The Transformation
Process and Circulation

There came a day for Harold when his avatar, Susan, woke up from a fitful sleep and just could not get going. He received the neurological reports coming into command central… all about malfunction: fatigue, aches, pains, sadness! He should have seen this coming. Having grown a little lax on the job, Harold had let his avatar spend more time in chairs, stop taking as many walks, discontinue her gym membership. How could he have done this? By this time in their relationship, he understood that blood flow to the outer reaches of the avatar unit was primary in maintaining good function, and movement activated the central pumping unit. Knowing that his avatar would only be able to tolerate gradual increases in her activity, he started by simply having her do some toe raises while she washed the dishes. Next, since she was currently working at a desk all day long, he had her set her watch alarm so that every hour she stood up and did a few knee bends. They started taking walks with friends, and while he wasn't sure whether it was the friends or the walks that made the difference, the mood register improved and the energy meter climbed.

Macrocirculation: Moving Feels Good

Writing this while sitting makes me feel a bit worried. Yikes! I need to stand up. I've had my booty in a chair for the past three hours, and I can feel my muffin top growing. Unfortunately, sitting is a new risk factor for dying early. It's not just that activity is good for you, lack of activity and increased sitting are risk factors for mortality. So stand on up, sweetie. How do we inject the fun here? Maybe a little chorus of "I Will Survive," adding a few toe raises, stretches, a few high knees. Seriously, I am doing this right now. Little movements matter. Remember the old abominable snowman putting one foot in front of the other? Moving more makes a difference.

—ᐩᐧᒧ— *Assignment* —ᐩᐧᒧ—

Right now, we're going to think about your posture. Get out of your chair and stretch your arms as high up as you can go. Take several deep breaths. Now change your posture and stand slumped over, allowing your body to fall onto your skeleton with less muscle tone. Next, take a breath and engage your muscles, rolling your shoulders back as you exhale slowly. Notice how energized you feel. Notice the difference between fully letting your bones support you and using posture that engages muscles.

That simple engagement translates to a difference in calories burned and muscle mass maintained. We all want to increase our metabolic rate (unfortunately because we usually want to eat more pizza), but increasing your metabolic rate through actively engaging muscles will help keep your muscles there! Active posture creates a sensation of power in your body. We are looking for ways to power up and this is a big one!

Fun and Speedy Exercise for Busy People

Easy. Fast. This is called 3-2-1 Done! And you're going to LOVE it!

3. Three minutes at 50%. Rest until your rate is down.

2. Two minutes at 75%. Rest until your heart rate is down.

1. 1 minute or (30 seconds) at 90%. Like running from a tiger! Then… can you guess? Yes, rest until your heart rate is down.

DONE!!!

As easy as that. You have 15 minutes? Great! (I know you do, so don't tell me you don't!) No costumes needed. Honestly, you don't even have to change into different shoes. You just have to get up out of that chair, put on some good music, and brace yourself. Have a little fun. I am so serious. One of my favorite things to do with clients is have them get up out of the chair and jump around the exam room for a couple minutes—yes, we do this together. First they think I'm nuts, then I tell them about the research that has been done proving the health benefits of simply standing up and doing some calisthenics.

If you prefer not to do calisthenics, please, by all means dance, boogie, jog in place, do burpees, wiggle, play Pokémon Go, do "the worm." Remember, we're all trying to avoid the seductive chair, and this short little exercise session, when done daily, could change your life.

So what's the research? Multiple controlled studies show that brief interval training is beneficial, particularly if you're out of shape. Some of these studies even revealed that this style of exercise can be as effective or more effective as longer bouts of cardiovascular training. A quick search on PubMed yields plenty of results on this. For instance, a study published in the March–April 2016 edition of *Journal of*

Cardiopulmonary Rehabilitation and Prevention evaluated 72 patients with ischemic heart disease, placing them in two groups: high-intensity interval training or moderate continuous training, both for eight weeks. Those patients who were placed into the high-intensity interval training group had improved increase in functional exercise capacity compared with moderate continuous training as well as a greater improvement in their quality of life without any increase in cardiovascular risk. (Jaureguizar KV 2016)

Maybe you don't have to slog on that jog to get your exercise out of the way. Yesterday my husband ran 27 miles. I think he's crazy—in a good way—but still....

I'm not the first person to talk about this, hopefully I will not be the last. Now promise me that you will to tell all your friends and neighbors about interval training, a wonderfully efficient way to exercise. Nice long cardio sessions and walks are wonderful too, but when you need to go ahead and finish already, the word on the street is **3-2-1 DONE!!**

Note: this protocol can be adjusted to whatever level of activity works for you—I have clients who do my 3-2-1 exercise seated in a wheelchair. And, of course, the universal disclaimer: if you have any health issues, don't begin a rigorous exercise program without the consent of your doctor, and if you have chest pain, please call 911.

Microcirculation

If you are an anesthesiologist, you think a lot about microcirculation. The rest of us? Not so much. Most of us have a vague notion of blood pressure, which is a measure of the pressure in our large arteries or our "macrocirculation." The microcirculation - movement of blood through the tiniest of capillaries feeds all the tissues of your body, bringing oxygen and nutrients, and removing waste products. A person's blood pressure might be okay, but if the blood is not moving well through the smaller capillaries it affects the health of all the surrounding cells. Hemodynamic coherence is the measurement of how well these are working in tandem. When someone has a heart attack and their heart stops, we must get it going again as soon as possible! During the time that a person's heart is not beating, CPR may be circulating blood in the big vessels, but the tiny vessels–the microcirculation and the body tissues are suffering. We have all heard stories of someone whose survival of a trauma led to an extended life with some part of their body (often their brain, because it is so sensitive) not working. This is because of lack of microcirculation. In order to recover enough to avoid the trip with the toe tag, they got back a blood pressure which implies reasonable macrocirculation. But you need both.

Microcirculation, for better or worse, is a significant factor in many phenomena: why high-intensity interval exercises are so effective, why we lose muscle mass and experience macular degeneration or poorer eyesight as we age... many chronic illnesses could improve with better microcirculation. These ideas are not revolutionary, after all; we all know that the optimizing macrocirculation or blood pressure can help these things. It's just that the poor capillaries get kind of ignored. And movement will always be the best ways to get your blood pumping; research has revealed possible physical methods to improve microcirculation. As reported in the October 2015 issue of the *Journal of Complementary and Integrative Medicine*, physical stimulation of the vasomotion of pre-capillary micro vessels (improved microcirculation) resulted in significant improvements on validated scales of sleep, pain, and quality of life over six weeks. (Bohn W 2013) Getting those blood cells moving is good medicine for your avatar!

—∿ι∕∽ *Assignment: Burst of Joy Exercise* —∿ι∕∽

Speaking of getting your blood pumping, little bursts of exercise are good for you. When you do something like take a quick, unexpected jog for 50 feet, your body wonders what the heck you are doing and how can it respond to make that activity easier and not such an insult. That's how our muscles get stronger and grow. We push them a little bit and that skooch of stress leads the body to beef itself up. I love the Burst of Joy exercise, because it's something that can be done anytime, anywhere, and it's more fun when you do it with a friend.

There are no limits as to what this can look like. It could be a jog in place, it can be a spontaneous dance, it could be quick sprint across the lawn. It might be something as simple as a head bob if you have just gotten out of surgery. Burst of joy implies opening your heart to the unbridled happiness of moving your body. Don't want to take a functioning body for granted; many of us will eventually find ourselves in a body that doesn't work quite right anymore. So even a little movement counts and gets you points toward leveling up. Have a hard time getting yourself to exercise? Well, let's make it a game.

You remember the drill:

- name your nemesis
- invite the bad guy to a challenge—your terms.
- arm your hero with qualities that will vanquish the enemy
- plan your battles in advance and practice
- keep a joyful score while battling

How do we turn exercise into a party? We invite friends. In Bellingham, we have a fantastic walking group that rotates its starting point among different businesses in the area and shares the dubious joy of walking in the Pacific Northwest weather. Putting a quick burst of joy into the walk here and there adds a little spice. A few jumping jacks, a few high knees—even little things can make a difference. We gain friends, we have the chance for community, and get to cash in on the idea that most things we don't really feel like doing become famously better with a buddy.

Ah, the accountability piece. Where is that scorecard, anyway? Are you someone who needs to answer to someone else to get things done? Maybe rebelling is a little more motivating for you, or perhaps your internal compass guides you to always do the right thing. For those who find that worrying about what others think affects their choices, using this personal knowledge can help you figure out the best way to motivate yourself. There is magic in having an accountability partner (a life coach, a friend, a family member, your doctor), someone who keeps tabs on you periodically and who you can send a quick message to saying what your goals are and what you've gotten done.

Chapter 11

The Transformation Process
and Environmental Alignment

Harold's avatar, Susan, created several new players called "babies" throughout their game. As fun as these new players were, they brought some environmental complications. With each new player, the environment grew more cluttered. At times, negotiating the avatar through the tight environment (obstacles scattered over the floor that could be dangerous to the structural integrity of the unit), and orchestrating the care of an exponentially large amount of stuff placed the avatar at risk and used a lot of neural networking and memory power, which compromised the ability to engage in the game worry-free. Harold slowly put a clutter-control system into place, freeing up brainpower as well as giving a sense of lightness and power to the unit.

Can You Say Clutter?

Let's talk about clutter control. You may already have a pristine, clutter-free home. For those of us who don't, part of healing is going to be letting go. We will be using the "toss ten today" technique. Just like it sounds, you need a bag, and maybe a friend who can help you—my friend Genia is a master at the toss. Maybe you have a buddy who can be your Genia. This is the friend who can look you in the eye and say, "Seriously, you're keeping that? You should give that away." Ten a day, give them away. If you haven't used it in a year, let it go. Don't forget to keep score! You need something that can make a fun sound as you toss things into the bag that goes to the thrift store. You don't have to stop at ten, but we want to do this every day until it's all better, so ten is a good number. Please do a victory dance. Please get out your theme song and play it very loud during purging! No one has done the study on cortisol levels and clutter, but I know for sure "tidy house" correlates with some pretty good feelings in my book.

One square foot at a time

What is your kitchen like? I can hear my husband laughing. Yes, I need a little work in this area. Happy to proudly claim that I am a work in progress. You are too, and that's alright. Converting your current environment into your Future You's dream home is a noble goal. I like to think of this as "one square foot at a time." You can combine this with the "toss ten today" technique.

The game is to take one square foot of space on a counter, floor, or shelf and wave your magic wand, transforming it to its future self. This feels so good. You will love yourself after you do this. Right now, put down this book and go find a square foot somewhere. Maybe you just want to find half of it. That's just fine. Make it beautiful. You may need a bag that will go to Goodwill. How do you make this fun and turn it into a game? Use your imagination. Put on some music. Use an application that will play a fun sound every time you press the button and put something into your bag. Play a fanfare at the end and chalk one up for your track record.

By this time, you probably have garnered a lot of points. What are you can do with those points? This is important to consider, what kind of treat will be in keeping with your future self? You need to have a plan to reward yourself for good deeds. We are not punishing here, only rewarding.

—ᐟᔓᐠ— *Assignment* —ᐟᔓᐠ—

Pick a square foot and go to town. It's going to feel so good when you're done.

Cabinet Purge

If you walk into your kitchen and have to drum up willpower to bypass the chips, you are just making it hard on yourself. Get rid of the foods that do not serve your body, making sure that you have healthy replacement. All you need is a big bag. Be ruthless. Remove the pseudo food. Give it to someone you know that isn't on a similar journey. If your cart at the grocery store always seems to somehow collect more processed food, use a grocery store that gives you the option of placing an online order and picking it up. Our Fred Meyer grocery store does this, and it's a time saver too!

Water and Air for Optimal Performance

Optimal avatar function requires pure water and air, free of toxicants. A good water filter is important in almost any type of dwelling. If you're a frequent soaker, then you might consider a filter on the water to your tub. A whole house water filter can be expensive, but if you are a home owner, this might be worth it. HEPA air filters make a huge difference, particularly if you have allergies, respiratory symptoms, and asthma.

Making sure your home is mold-free and that there is no standing water helps minimize potential exposure to toxic mold. Some people's bodies tolerate mold exposure without much problem; their ability to process and continue to function well makes them resilient. Others who have had multiple exposures to toxins, chronic viral infections, poor diet, or who are genetically predisposed to problems with biotransformation (the natural way that we process the garbage our body does not want or need) might take one big whiff of black mold and feel very, very bad. Some folks can live with a mouthful of mercury amalgam fillings, no problem. Some folks with a mouthful of mercury amalgams feel terrible and have no idea why. It has to do with their ability for their cells to be exposed to mercury and still keep functioning.

Have you ever been to a water park with one of those huge buckets that is slowly filling until it all spills out? Think of your body like that in terms of its ability to manage exposures over your lifetime. If various substances that could be toxic keep adding up and keep drip, drip, dripping into your bucket, there comes a point where normal functions don't function normally. Your amazing body is created with the ability to clear a myriad of compounds that would otherwise make us sick. But a long list of things make that killer cleaner upper machinery malfunction or even break…. Drip, drip, drip…. Too much of the bad stuff, the bucket spills over and you feel like crap.

Time to return to living more like our grandparents did, avoiding processed foods that have ingredients that you cannot pronounce, being careful with cleaners, choosing green and environmentally sound products. An infamous study performed in 2004 and spearheaded by the Environmental Working Group looked at the umbilical cord blood, collected by the Red Cross, from 10 newborn babies. A total of 287 chemicals were isolated from babies *who had not even been out of the womb*. This was the first time that 209 of these compounds had ever been identified in cord blood. 180 of these compounds are known to cause cancer in humans and animals, 217 create toxicity in the nervous system, and 208 can cause birth defects or abnormal development and animal tests. Chemicals we allowed to be used in products, services, the environment, and our body are going to affect us and our children.

How can we turn detox into a game? Take heart, start wherever you are. It's okay if you are immersed in a world of products, potions, cleaners, toxic people and relationships, automatic thoughts, exposures—that gives you more to work with. Set a timer and make a list. How many toxic exposures can you identify in your life? Play some fun music while you make this list. Get as many things written down as you possibly can.

Inventory of toxic exposures: check. Basic principle here, we are trying to increase the good and decrease the bad. Toxic exposures = bad. You have your hit list now. You have several choices and how to deal with items on your hit list.

- eliminate
- trade up
- redefine/evolve
- postpone

Take your list and decide which action is most appropriate for each item. Eliminating can be life-giving. Feels so good to let go sometimes. Trading up can work for products and relationships. Redefining is an inner job; sometimes environments, people, or memories hold powerful influence over our state of mind, and that interpretation can be shifted through intention. Right now we're just figuring out what approach would be best for each of these mangy critters; so don't fret if you're not sure how to go about the redefinition. Postponing? Decide to not decide right now. That's a-okay! Remember, this is a marathon, not a sprint.

Now that you have gone through your list and decided how you might approach each item, let's just pick one. Pick an easy one. It's time to create a track record. The steps are the same:

- bestow unto the toxin a game name
- challenge the nemesis to come onto your court—your terms
- arm your hero
- visualize the battle in advance
- battle with scorecard in hand!

Chapter 12

The Transformation
Process and Connection

Synchronization: Strengthening the Dream Team Bonds

Support for your quest can come from many different places, and developing a dream team can move you toward your goals faster. During your personal visioning exercise, one of the tasks was to imagine the people you will be spending time with. Some may be folks you already know, some may be people with qualities that you want to emulate or that might complete your inner circle. In this part of the game, the goal is identifying and developing healthy relationships with those who take you to your higher self. We tend to take on characteristics of the few people with whom we spend the most time.

Synchronization is matching up what's going on with your body with the person with whom you are spending time. Research shows that during gameplay, we start to synchronize with them on a physical level. Our heart rates and breathing match more closely, our body gestures and posture tends to mirror our gaming partner. This synchrony correlates with a bond of empathy and understanding. Hence the value in kids visiting and playing board games with people in nursing homes. A person can benefit from synchronizing with someone through actions as simple as matching pace and step while walking together, intentionally breathing at a similar rate with someone else, singing a song together, swaying to a musical beat in synchronicity. (Valdesolo P 2011) Every little positive connection contributes to a shift toward your amazing transformation.

—✦— *Assignment* —✦—

Notice synchrony between people in your environment, and intentionally create this with another person when you are needing a boost. It could be as simple as assuming a similar position or breathing at the same time.

Connection: Spending Time with People You Enjoy Makes You Healthier

A 2010 meta-analysis evaluated multiple research studies that looked at how social connections affect people's health, finding that a lack of social connectivity was a risk factor for illness. It's not just that being connected with friends and family and those who share common interests is beneficial; the lack of community connection actually makes diseases worse. (Tanskanen J 2016) Part of the game of revolutionizing your health necessitates intentionally hanging out with someone or a group of people that you enjoy. What great news!

Sometimes we have to look for that group—it may be that you are isolated, have few friends, or don't relate to people in your area. It may be that your friends and loved ones have died and you are feeling alone. We can turn the hunt for buddies into a bit of a game also. Many of us tend to slowly isolate as we age, or as we are in immersed in the "busyness" of daily life. The evening time might become the only moment of the day when you feel like you can catch your breath. There are many more ways to socialize besides attending a party or getting together. Here are some ideas about how you can start to squeeze community into a life that has no apparent room for community:

- Take a group lesson for a new hobby—you always wanted to learn to do that, right?
- Find a spiritual community of like-minded people.
- Find a way to volunteer for a good cause.
- Invite someone to tea.
- Play an online game such as Candy Crush Saga, Words with Friends, online Scrabble, or Chess.
- Share a personal gift such as the ability to cook with a friend.
- Find someone you can help somehow.
- Send an encouraging text.
- Write a letter to an old friend or get a pen pal.
- Play family games or charades.

I'm sure you can think of many more ways to add community into your life. We are social beings that require the giving and receiving of love for optimal health. Certain people will start to filter out and become sources of strength and support. These are the entities (I say entities because sometimes it is our pets) who will become part of your posse.

Connection: Do You Need to Cut the Cord?

This isn't a relationship book. Lots of those out there. This is a revelation book. On your toxic list, are there people? Challenging relationships can create the richest fodder for emotional and spiritual growth, and how we deal with them depends on the importance of the relationship, our energy, and our time. Recognizing that a relationship is sucking your everlasting soul is the first step, just like recognizing toxic thoughts. When looking at options for dealing with toxic exposures—eliminate, trade up, redefine, and postpone—I suggest using one of the first three when it comes to relationships. Notice, too, that toxic relationship stress often comes from self-talk around the relationship, believing someone else's negative script, and/or placing unreasonable pressure on oneself within the relationship. My husband likes to say, "Never let the instability of others ruin your day." Words to live by. We are all given "gifts" by our families, and those "gifts" often require a good therapist for resolution. Why don't they teach good coping and communication skills in elementary school? Go figure.

In case you haven't realized this, people learn how to deal with adversity through watching their families, sometimes picking up "tips and tricks" that totally do not work in the process. (Remember the lessons that Harold figured out as he puzzled over the behaviors of his original gaming group!) Those tips and tricks go on to be our coping mechanisms that our spouses and loved ones have to suffer through until we realize that we have been duped and sent down a wrong corridor in our game of life. For instance, if that temper tantrum always got somebody their way through elementary school, then middle school, then high school, then college, then... guess what? They will continue doing that to get their way—but now with an adult spin. The relationship's value determines the amount of effort one should put into the redefinition/ evolution option. Sometimes we need a spouse-ectomy, a job-ectomy, a friend-ectomy; hard to say, but true.

If elimination or trading up is not the answer for the particular relationship in question, evolve using a game. Research shows that playing games together increases empathy, improves intergenerational relations, and increases cooperation. Playing a relationship-boosting game and winning together could mean reclaiming and rekindling the romance of a lifetime. My favorite piece of marital gaming advice is the "do-over," so I must include it here. Any time there's an uncomfortable, bad, or nasty exchange between two people who beneath the exchange have a loving relationship, the "do-over" game is an amazing tool. Any person can call a do-over. You rewind the tape, go back to the physical spot where the exchange started and do it again. Say things a little differently, choose your words more carefully, think about the other person's point of view and make a new memory. Keeping score makes it into a game; I suggest keeping track of how many do-overs you do in a day, in a week. The more the better. It means you are thinking about how you engage your partner, your kid, your friend. Notice the difference between the way your body feels after the initial interaction and after the do-over. It's like magic.

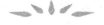

Conclusion

Feel Good Again...and Again

A Spectacular Merry-Go-Round

Throughout this book, our focus has been on how you can motivate yourself to do the things that you want to do and make the changes you would like to make by using gaming strategies to make it fun. I'd like to tell you that the newness of this perspective will last forever, but even that is going to get old. The new toy gets a little rusty, the paint chips off. We get a little tired of going to that exercise class, and, well, the Kung Fu was fun for a bit, now the couch looks a little better.

The second part of maintaining a state of evolution is creating a cycle. Similar to creating balance in your sympathetic and parasympathetic nervous system, we want to create balance through an "effort and enjoy" cycle. Do you know anyone who always needs to have a new project? Someone who, just as soon as they finish the last project, is on to the next one and never takes a breath? (Yes, family, I know what you are thinking.) Classic recipe for burnout. I invite you to engage in a cycle that you will re-create every two to three months:

- Initially rediscovering yourself and reinventing yourself
- Booting the bad
- Boosting the positive
- Gaining power and momentum
- Focusing on your blissful balance
- Reassessing
- Enjoy, ingrain, solidify what you've done over the past several weeks
- Then begin again

Rediscovery and Reinvention

As you plan your reinvention, I would like you to imagine that you are the "driver" of the avatar that is your body. See if you can possibly remove the charge and judgment, let go of the emotion of your personal issues, and think of your mind as the player of the game, the one in the little control room who's trying to level up their avatar. The first phase of the cycle involves holding up the mirror: introspection, evaluation, truly understanding, appreciating the unique circumstances of your avatar. If only you had realized this when you were a kid, or a teenager, that your big job actually is proper care and maintenance of the avatar so it can perform well for you, you can enjoy yourself in the process, and you can get higher in the game.

Interesting to think of how many strata of engagement there might be as we play. What gaming level do you think folks like Abraham Lincoln, Mother Teresa, Gandhi, Thomas Jefferson, or Martin Luther King achieved? Do we perform better in the game and level up faster if we play for other people and try and affect their game in positive ways?

If we assume that taking care of our avatar gives us points, what does it mean to our trajectory in the game when we ignore self-care?

The first phase of your every cycle is recording where you are in this moment. Take the tests, record your score, do a couple of days of intense journaling. This is going to yield a big list of your good points, your bad points, things you want to change, things you love, all your habits. In your mind, I want you to go through that exercise of visually rolling up all these documents, seeing them transform into the most spectacular butterfly you have ever seen. At this point, it is important to complete the Feel Good Again Questionnaire. You might not be able to see improvement unless you're tracking yourself.

Next we have the reinvention. The amazing butterfly must be quantified. Time to get in touch with your hopes, dreams, aspirations for the health of your mind, body, spirit, and material manifestations. Crystal clear visioning exercise with no holds barred. Remove limits and catapult yourself to your future. Targets tend to shift as we grow and change. A plane on a trip across the country has to continually redirect, and sometimes gets rerouted. What's nice about this cycle is you have a chance to reinvent yourself every two to three months. It's like a rebirth, a chance to start over. When you have a clear picture, including as many juicy details as you can possibly squeeze into your head, then it's time to create your game for the month. We all have many compartments in our lives: work, health, spirituality, family, community, relationships, friends, and politics. You get what I mean. This gives multiple possibilities in terms of what you want to work on.

What is the difference between here and there? What are the skills required for your avatar to gain in order to become Future You? What self-disciplines will be developed by that time? Each cycle, you will make a flowchart that shows the steps your avatar will go through in order to level up to those goals. Say, for instance, you have diabetes and weight challenges and have tried many times to lose weight unsuccessfully, but have been thwarted by cravings and pain when you exercise, lack of time, and a feeling of discomfort when you've started to lose weight as though you had lost a little bit of your "protective shield." The long-term goal might be to reverse the diabetes and lose the weight, but there are many worthwhile steps and lessons in between here and there. It could involve environmental change, like a shift in foods you are eating, inner work involving self-love, increasing activity, or even finding a new job. If you can envision the path with as much detail as possible, mapping your quest is easy. As an aside, some things in our quest require clerical work, getting on the phone, talking to someone, signing up for something. These sorts of tasks should not be ignored if they stand between you and Future You. They go on your to-do list.

Some people try and change it all in one fell swoop. In my experience, this is difficult to maintain. You can eat an elephant one little bite at a time. So my suggestion would be to select one to four areas in which you would like to make a shift, craft a quest, and just work on the next step in these areas. Some people would prefer to identify several steps in one area, and that is fine. Small little changes are more likely to stick for most people.

Quest Creation

Recall the steps to quest creation.

Step 1. **Check In: current state of health (Feel Good Again questionnaire)**

Step 2. **Take Stock: of where I am today (The Mirror)**

Step 3. **Time Travel: to meet my future self**

Step 4: **Draw the Map: design the journey between here and there**

Another way to think of quest creation is to consider how you can…

- Increase the good—habits, people, environment, thoughts, activities
- Decrease the bad—remove obstacles that stand between current and Future You
- Achieve balance in that area

In terms of goal-setting and achievement, this program places most value on focusing on regular daily activity and playing the game, keeping score in your day-to-day routines. You only work on the next step…one little thing at a time. Once you create the road map you can put it away and focus on a single improvement. (It would be overwhelming to keep looking at that!) We hold our gaze on the outcome and just do the next step.

The measure of success is tracked through monthly snapshots using the Feel Good Again Questionnaire. Most people don't notice little day-to-day changes; the magic is in the monthly measurement, revealing the shifts. Generally six weeks gives people a substantial amount of change, improvement in their feelings of self-efficacy (that means they feel like they can do something about their health), symptoms, mood, and energy level. Include:

- Monthly measurement of progress. Seriously, you will not think this works if you do not measure it.
- Five minutes to plan out your day, every day.
- Simple daily scorekeeping using an application or a pencil. The simpler the better.
- Daily visualization of success while in a meditative state.

- Take the time to turn it into a game. If you don't turn it into a game, you are using old ways to muscle yourself into doing something.

If you continue to follow the Feel Good Again Plan with a regular assessment, challenge creation, and built-in "bask in the glory of my new habits" time (to maintain and cement down what works), you'll find yourself moving closer to the future vision you cast. As you evolve, remember that everybody is a work in progress, each of us with potential beyond our imagination. In order to keep winding our way up the ladder of personal growth, we must learn to be compassionate to ourselves and others, and look for the positive, even when it's difficult to see.

Have fun and keep your eyes on the prize!

Bibliography

Banyan, Carl. 2003. *The Secret Language of Feelings*. Tustin: Banyan Hypnosis Center for Training and Services, Inc.

Bohn W, Hess L, Burger R. 2013. "The effects of the "physical BEMER® vascular therapy", a method for the physical stimulation of the vasomotion of precapillary microvessels in case of impaired microcirculation, on sleep, pain and quality of life of patients with different clinical picture." *Journal of complementary and integrative medicine* 2013;10(Suppl):S5-12, S5-13.

Christakis NA, Fowler JH. 2007. "The spread of obesity in a large social network over 32 years." *New England Journal of Medicine* Jul 26;357(4):370-9.

Duhig, Charles. 2014. *The Power of Habit*. New York: Random House Trade Paperbacks.

—. 2014. *The Power of Habit*. New York: Random House Trade Paperbacks.

Hottenrott K, Hoos O, Esperer HD. 2006. "Heart rate variability and physical exercise. Current status." *Herz* Sep;31(6):544-52.

Jaureguizar KV, Vicente-Campos D, Bautista LR, de la Peña CH, Gómez MJ, Rueda MJ, Fernández Mahillo I. 2016. "Effect of High-Intensity Interval Versus Continuous Exercise Training on Functional Capacity and Quality of Life in Patients With Coronary Artery Disease: A RANDOMIZED CLINICAL TRIAL." *Journal of cardiopulmonary rehabilitation and prevention* Mar-Apr;36(2):96-105.

JG, Dong. 2106. "The role of heart rate variability in sports physiology." *Experimental and Therapeutic Medicine* May;11(5):1531-1536.

McGonigal, J. 2015. *Super Better*. New York: Penguin Press.

Mirmiran P, Bahadoran Z, Khalili Moghadam S, Zadeh Vakili A, Azizi F. 2016. "A Prospective Study of Different Types of Dietary Fiber and Risk of Cardiovascular Disease: Tehran Lipid and Glucose Study." *Nutrients* Nov 7;8(11).

Moss, Simon A, Timothy C Skinner, Nektarios Alexi, and Samuel G Wilson. September 22, 2016. "Look into the crystal ball: Can vivid images of the future enhance physical health?" *J Health Psycho.*

Pham, Lien B, Taylor, Shelley E. Feb1999 Volume 25 No. 2. "From Thought to Action: Effects of Process-Versus Outcome-Based Mental Simulations on Performance." *Pers Soc Psychol Bull* 250-260.

Sawka KJ, McCormack GR, Nettel-Aguirre A, Swanson K. 2015. "Associations between aspects of friendship networks and dietary behavior in youth: Findings from a systematized review." *Eating Behaviors* Aug;18:7-15.

Sirois FM, Wood AM. 2016. "Gratitude Uniquely Predicts Lower Depression in Chronic Illness Populations: A Longitudinal Study of Inflammatory Bowel Disease and Arthritis." *Health Psychology.*

Stellar JE, John-Henderson N, Anderson CL, Gordon AM, McNeil GD, Keltner D. 2015. "Positive affect and markers of inflammation: discrete positive emotions predict lower levels of inflammatory cytokines." *Emotion* Apr;15(2):129-33.

Tanskanen J, Anttila T. 2016. "A Prospective Study of Social Isolation, Loneliness, and Mortality in Finland." *American Journal of public health* Nov;106(11):2042-2048.

Valdesolo P, Desteno D. 2011. "Synchrony and the social tuning of compassion." *Emotion* Apr;11(2):262-6.

Watt RG, Heilmann A1, Sabbah W, Newton T, Chandola T, Aida J, Sheiham A, Marmot M, Kawachi I, Tsakos G. 2014. "Social relationships and health related behaviors among older US adults." *BMC Public Health* May 30;14:533.

Appendix

Taking Stock Questionnaire Links
Feel Good Again Questionnaire (go to my website):
www.sunnygmd.com/feel-good-again-book-resources/

For those with anxiety:
www.thecalculator.co/health/Generalized-Anxiety-Disorder-GAD-7-Calculator-802.html

For those with depression, depressive symptoms, or mood challenges:
www.mdcalc.com/phq-9-patient-health-questionnaire-9/

Values in Action Questionnaire:
www.viacharacter.org/www/Character-Strengths-Survey

Resources for Working with Your Genetics:

23andMe is an online service you can use to obtain a copy of your genetics:

www.23andme.com/

Promethease is a literature retrieval system that builds a personal DNA report based on connecting a file of DNA genotypes to the scientific findings cited in SNPedia.

Biomedical researchers, healthcare practitioners and customers of DNA testing services (such as 23andMe, Ancestry.com, FamilyTreeDNA, etc.) use Promethease to retrieve information published about their DNA variations. Most reports cost $5 and are produced in under 10 minutes. Much larger data files (such as imputed full genomes from dna.land) cost $10 and have increased runtime.

www.promethease.com/

For information which focuses on your variations that relate to methylation and bio transformation:

www.knowyourgenetics.com/

Supplement Recommendations

These are very basic supplement recommendations. Remember to find a supplement company that is GMP (Good Manufacturing Practices) certified. It is important to speak with your healthcare provider regarding the best practices for you.

- Multivitamin/multi-mineral supplement.
- Vitamin D3 1000 international units daily. Levels need to be checked to determine that you're not getting too much or too little. Work with your provider to get your levels within recommended range. See appendix for optimal values.
- Omega-3 fatty acids or fish oil/krill oil supplement. I recommend 2000 mg for the average person. Those with inflammatory and

autoimmune issues may benefit from a higher dose; speak with your health care provider about dosing recommendations.

- B complex vitamin daily.
- Daily probiotic 25 Billion CFUs or fermented foods (like kombucha, sauerkraut, pickled veggies, kimchi) daily.

Reader Resources

Connect to Dr. Linda (Sunny) Goggin:
Website: www.lindagogginmd.com/
Facebook page:
    Dr. Goggin: www.facebook.com/sunnygmd/
    Feel Good Again Book Club: www.facebook.com/2monthphoenix/
Twitter: twitter.com/lindagogginmd/
Community forum: www.sunnygmd.com/community-forum/? p=%3F
Sunny's Victory Dance: www.sunnygmd.com/sunnys-victory-dance/
    LinkedIn: www.linkedin.com/in/linda-goggin-611164116

Gaming Applications:
    Habitica: www.youtube.com/watch? v=hgdeJnSili0

Jane McGonigal PhD Ted Talk about SuperBetter game:
    www.youtube.com/watch? v=lfBpsV1Hwqs

Functional Medicine Information:
www.functionalmedicine.org/

Environmental Working Group Dirty Dozen and Clean Fifteen:
www.ewg.org/foodnews/dirty_dozen_list.php

PubMed
www.ncbi.nlm.nih.gov/pubmed/

Acknowledgments

My Book Posse

Maggie McReynolds, thank you for your fantastic editing, believing in me, and helping me to bring my message to the world. Lots of hugs! You're the best editor a gal could ask for!

Angela Lauria, thank you for putting together a wonderful program that allowed me to make my dream come true of writing a book that matters!

Order of the Quill sisters, thank you for your encouragement as we walk this path together. So much more fun with friends!

To the Morgan James Publishing team: Special thanks to David Hancock, CEO & Founder for believing in me and my message. To my Author Relations Manager, Margo Toulouse, thanks for making the process seamless and easy. Many more thanks to everyone else, but especially Jim Howard, Bethany Marshall, and Nickcole Watkins.

My Home Posse

Charlie, Zoe, and Henry Goggin, you guys were also patient with me when I disappeared into the nook. Thank you for supporting me; I'm the luckiest mom ever! I hope one day you will have fun reading this book; it is really written for you!

Colin Goggin, thanks for your love and support as this book came together. You made it possible by being so patient and kind. Thanks for always shining the beacon of evidenced-based medicine.

My Work Posse

Pamela Wible, MD, I would never have written this book if I had not stumbled across your wonderful group. Taking the plunge into my own practice was scary, but I am a different person and a better doctor because of it.

Tom Malterre, thanks for being such a great friend and inspiration.

Maureen Skipton and Miqua Corrigan, thank you so much for being amazing coaches!

Jesse Larsen, thank you for stepping up and helping me in ways I didn't even know I needed! You're awesome!

Robi Hawley, thanks for all your amazing know-how and support!

The Institute for Functional Medicine, thanks for being the guiding light to those of us who knew there was something more to medicine than checking off boxes.

All my clients, every day I'm inspired by you and your journeys. Thank you for putting trust in me to help.

I'm sure there are others that should be included—I feel so grateful to all the wonderful influences in my life. Thank you!

About the Author

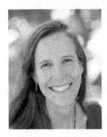

Linda Goggin MD, affectionately known as "Sunny" to those around her, considers putting the "fun" into Functional Medicine her prime objective. During a time when everyone is giving advice on "what" to do, Sunny wants to help people with the "how." Starting out as a hospital volunteer, then as a nurse's aide, then as a registered nurse, Dr. Goggin went to medical school at Emory University in Atlanta, Georgia. After all these years, she still would do it again in a heartbeat.

During her career Dr. Goggin has explored several roles in medicine, including hospitalist, directing a Health Department in rural North Carolina, being a "country doc"—one minute in the emergency room and the next minute in the clinic or hospital—and working in a busy suburban family practice clinic. After moving from NC to Bellingham,

WA, she found her love affair with medicine reignited on discovering and implementing the Functional Medicine Model in her personal medical practice.

Today, Dr. Goggin hones her ability to motivate and guide daily by attempting to subtly manipulate her husband and three kids, as well as caring for patients at Bellingham Functional Medicine, where she collaborates with Functional Nutritionist powerhouse and author Tom Malterre, MS, CN (The Elimination Diet, Nourishing Meals). She is also the owner and medical director of Ideal Health Bellingham, which provides medical weight loss guidance and primary care.

A pioneer on the edge of medicine, Dr. Goggin created the first Direct Primary Care Practice in Bellingham, where she remains passionate about empowering clients to claim their health vision and race toward it with wild abandon. She thinks creating health is a fantastically cool game once you figure out where to aim your arrow, point, and shoot. So get out your bow and let's go!

Thank You

Thank you so much for taking the time to read Feel Good Again. I hope that it gives you a new perspective on how to shift your health... a little bit more joy, a little bit more fun, and empowerment to make big changes.

Race to my website and download your FREE thank you video series and handy Feel Good Again Tool Kit!

Video Download
www.sunnygmd.com/feel-good-again-book-resources/feel-good-again-...e-video-download/

Tool Kit Download
www.sunnygmd.com/feel-good-again-book-resources/

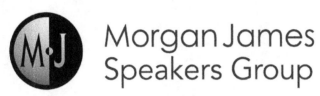

Morgan James
Speakers Group

www.TheMorganJamesSpeakersGroup.com

We connect Morgan James published
authors with live and online events
and audiences whom will benefit
from their expertise.

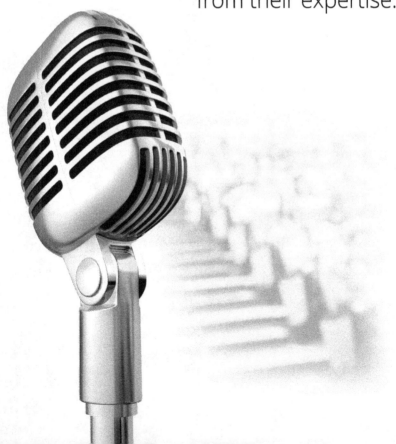

Morgan James makes all of our titles available
through the Library for All Charity Organization.

www.LibraryForAll.org